OZEMPIC REVOLUTION

THE ESSENTIAL GUIDE TO MANAGING DIABETES AND LOSING WEIGHT

Dr. Jaox Clement Jackie

Disclaimer:

The information provided here is for general informational purposes only and is not intended to be a substitute for professional medical advice, diagnosis, or treatment. Always seek the advice of your physician or other qualified health provider with any questions you may have regarding a medical condition.

The content in this information does not constitute medical advice, and reliance on any information provided by this source is solely at your own risk. The author and publisher of this content are not medical professionals, and the content should not be considered as medical consultation.

Information about medications, including Ozempic, is subject to change, and developments in medical research may impact the information provided. Always consult your healthcare provider for the most current and personalized advice regarding your specific health situation and the use of any medication.

The author and publisher disclaim any liability for any adverse effects or consequences resulting from the use of the information provided here. Any mention of specific medications, brands, or medical treatments does not constitute an endorsement, and individual responses to medication may vary.

It is crucial to follow your healthcare provider's advice, prescription, and instructions when using any medication, including Ozempic. Do not disregard professional medical advice or delay seeking it based on information provided in this content.

By accessing and using this information, you acknowledge and agree to the terms of this disclaimer.

Table of Contents

CHAPTER ELEVEN
Conclusion

11.1 Summary of Key Points
11.2 Future Developments

8

CHAPTER ONE

Introduction to Ozempic

1.1 What is Ozempic?

Ozempic is the brand name of the drug semaglutide, which belongs to a class of drugs called glucagon-like peptide-1 (GLP-1) receptor agonists. It is used to treat type 2 diabetes in adults by helping to lower blood sugar levels. Ozempic works by mimicking the action of GLP-1, a hormone produced in the intestine that stimulates insulin release from the pancreas and reduces glucose production in the liver. This helps regulate blood sugar levels after meals and throughout the day. In addition to lowering blood sugar levels, Ozempic may also promote weight loss and have cardiovascular and renal benefits in certain people with type 2 diabetes. It is administered once a week as a subcutaneous injection and is usually used in combination with diet and exercise to improve blood sugar control. As with any medicine, it is important to use Ozempic under a doctor's supervision.

1.2 Drug Overview

Ozempic (semaglutide) is a medicine used to treat type 2 diabetes. It belongs to the class of so-called glucagon-like peptide-1 receptor agonists (GLP-1 RA).

Here's a summary of what this medication does:

Mechanism of action: Ozempic works by mimicking the effects of the natural hormone GLP-1. It stimulates the GLP-1 receptors in the pancreas, resulting in increased insulin secretion and decreased glucagon secretion. This helps lower blood sugar levels in people with type 2 diabetes by improving insulin sensitivity and decreasing glucose production in the liver.

Administration: Ozempic is administered by subcutaneous injection once a week. The medication comes in a pre-filled pen so patients can self-administer it in the comfort of their own home. **Efficacy:** Clinical studies have shown that Ozempic is effective in lowering blood glucose levels in people with type 2 diabetes. It has also been associated with weight loss in many patients, making it a valuable option for individuals who need to improve both glycemic control and weight management.

Dosage: The recommended starting dose of Ozempic is typically 0.25 mg once weekly, which may be increased to 0.5 mg after 4 weeks depending on individual response. Some patients may benefit from a further increase to 1 mg once weekly, but may require a lower dose due to tolerability or other factors.

Side Effects: Common side effects of Ozempic include nausea, vomiting, diarrhea, and abdominal pain, especially when treatment is initiated or the dose is increased. These side effects usually improve over time as your body gets used to the medication. Serious side effects, such as pancreatitis or allergic reactions, are rare but can occur.

Precautions: Ozempic should be used with caution in people with a history of pancreatitis, thyroid disease, or kidney problems. It is important that your medical staff evaluate your medical history and monitor you regularly during treatment.

Benefits beyond blood sugar control: In addition to its primary role in lowering blood sugar levels, Ozempic has been shown to have potential cardiovascular health benefits. Clinical studies have shown that patients treated with Ozempic have a reduced risk of heart attack, stroke, and cardiovascular death.

1.3 How does Ozempic work?

Ozempic (semaglutide) works primarily by mimicking the effects of a hormone called glucagon-like peptide-1 (GLP-1) that is produced naturally in the body. Here is a detailed explanation of how Ozempic works:

GLP-1 receptor agonist: Ozempic belongs to a class of drugs known as GLP-1 receptor agonists. These drugs activate GLP-1 receptors, which are found in various tissues throughout the body, including the pancreas, liver, stomach, and brain.

Stimulation of insulin secretion: One of the most important effects of GLP-1 is to stimulate insulin secretion from the pancreas in response to rising blood glucose levels. When blood sugar levels rise after a meal, GLP-1 is released from specialized cells in the intestine. Ozempic increases insulin secretion by activating GLP-1 receptors on beta cells in the pancreas. Insulin promotes glucose absorption into cells, lowering blood sugar levels.

Inhibition of glucagon release: In addition to stimulating insulin release, GLP-1 also inhibits the release of another hormone called glucagon. Glucagon normally increases blood sugar levels by promoting the release of stored glucose from the liver. By reducing the release of glucagon, Ozempic reduces the amount of glucose produced in the liver, further helping to control blood sugar levels.

Delayed Gastric Emptying: GLP-1 receptors are also found in the stomach and help regulate gastric emptying. When Ozempic activates these receptors, it slows down the rate at which food passes through the digestive system. This delayed gastric emptying makes you feel full or satisfied, reducing food intake and helping with weight loss.

Effects on the Central Nervous System:
GLP-1 receptors are also found in the brain and play a role in regulating appetite and food intake. Ozempic reduces appetite and cravings by activating these receptors in the brain, thereby supporting weight loss.

1.4 Mechanism of Action

Ozempic (semaglutide) mechanism of action revolves around its role as a glucagon-like peptide-1 receptor agonist (GLP-1). Here is a detailed explanation:

Activation of GLP-1 receptors: Ozempic binds to and activates GLP-1 receptors found on various cells throughout the body, including pancreatic beta cells, liver cells, stomach cells, and neurons in the brain.

Stimulation of insulin secretion: Ozempic stimulates insulin secretion by activating GLP-1 receptors on pancreatic beta cells. Insulin is a hormone responsible for absorbing glucose from the bloodstream into cells, where it can be used to produce energy or store for later use. By increasing insulin secretion, Ozempic helps lower blood sugar levels, especially after meals, when blood sugar levels are likely to rise.

Inhibition of glucagon release: Ozempic also inhibits the release of glucagon, another hormone produced by the pancreas. Glucagon increases blood sugar levels by promoting the release of stored glucose from the liver into the bloodstream. By reducing the release of glucagon, Ozempic reduces glucose production in the liver, further helping to regulate blood sugar levels.

Delayed gastric emptying: Ozempic's activation of GLP-1 receptors in the stomach slows the rate at which food passes through the digestive system. This delayed gastric emptying makes you feel full, which may reduce food intake and lead to weight loss.
Appetite suppressant: GLP-1 receptors in the brain are involved in regulating appetite and food intake. By activating these receptors in specific regions of the brain, Ozempic reduces appetite and cravings, thereby supporting weight loss.

Cardiovascular Effects: Ozempic has shown potential benefits for cardiovascular health beyond its effects on glycemic control and weight management. Clinical studies have shown that patients treated with Ozempic have a reduced risk of serious cardiovascular events, including heart attack, stroke, and cardiovascular death.

Overall, Ozempic's mechanism of action involves multiple pathways that contribute to improved glycemic control, weight loss, and potential cardiovascular benefits in patients with type 2 diabetes. By targeting the GLP-1 receptor, Ozempic addresses an important aspect of diabetes treatment and may help reduce the risk of diabetes-related complications.

1.5 Benefits of Ozempic

Ozempic (semaglutide) offers several benefits to people with type 2 diabetes. Some of the main benefits include:

Improved glycemic control: Ozempic helps lower blood glucose levels by stimulating insulin secretion and inhibiting glucagon secretion. By mimicking the action of the hormone GLP-1, Ozempic promotes more effective glucose utilization by cells and reduces glucose production by the liver. This improves overall glycemic control, as evidenced by lower hemoglobin A1c (HbA1c) levels, which reflect average blood glucose levels over time.

Weight loss: Many people with type 2 diabetes suffer from overweight or obesity, which can worsen insulin resistance and make glycemic control more difficult. One notable benefit of Ozempic is its association with weight loss. Ozempic helps you lose weight and maintain that weight over the long term by slowing stomach emptying, suppressing appetite, and promoting feelings of fullness. This weight loss helps improve insulin sensitivity and overall metabolic health.

Cardiovascular Benefits: Clinical studies have demonstrated potential cardiovascular benefits associated with Ozempic treatment. These benefits include a reduced risk of serious cardiovascular events, such as heart attack, stroke, and cardiovascular death. The exact mechanisms underlying these cardiovascular benefits are not yet fully understood but may include improvements in vascular function, inflammation and other cardiovascular risk factors.

Ease of administration: Ozempic is administered by subcutaneous injection once weekly. The drug comes in a prefilled pen, allowing patients to self-administer it in the comfort of their own home. This once-weekly administration schedule simplifies treatment and may improve compliance compared to medications that must be administered daily.

Potential renal protection: Emerging evidence suggests that GLP-1 receptor agonists, including Ozempic, may have beneficial effects on renal function and may help reduce the risk of kidney disease progression in patients with type 2 diabetes. Further studies are needed to fully elucidate the renal protective effects of Ozempic and other GLP-1 agonists.

Safety Profile: Ozempic has demonstrated a generally favorable safety profile in clinical studies. Common side effects include nausea, vomiting, diarrhea, and abdominal pain, especially when treatment is initiated or doses are increased. Serious side effects, such as pancreatitis and allergic reactions, are rare but can occur and require monitoring by a healthcare professional.

Overall, Ozempic offers many benefits beyond glycemic control, including weight loss, potential cardiovascular protection, and convenience of administration. These benefits make it a valuable treatment option for people with type 2 diabetes, especially those who may benefit from improved metabolic and cardiovascular health. As with any medication, it is important that patients discuss the potential benefits and risks of Ozempic with their doctor to determine if Ozempic is the right choice for them.

1.6 Benefits of Diabetes Treatment

Ozempic (semaglutide) offers several benefits in diabetes treatment, making it a valuable treatment option for people with type 2 diabetes. Some of the key benefits include:

Effective glycemic control: One of the main benefits of Ozempic is its ability to effectively lower blood glucose levels. As a glucagon-like peptide-1 receptor agonist (GLP-1), Ozempic controls blood glucose levels throughout the day by stimulating insulin secretion and inhibiting glucagon secretion. By improving glycemic control, Ozempic may reduce the risk of complications associated with hyperglycemia, such as diabetic neuropathy, retinopathy, and nephropathy.

Weight loss: Many people with type 2 diabetes are overweight or obese, which can worsen insulin resistance and make glycemic control more difficult. Ozempic has been shown to be effective in weight loss in clinical studies, making it an attractive option for people who need to control both their blood sugar and weight. Ozempic's weight loss effect is thought to be due to delayed gastric emptying, reduced food intake, and increased satiety.

Cardiovascular benefits: Clinical studies have demonstrated potential cardiovascular benefits associated with Ozempic treatment. These benefits include a reduced risk of serious cardiovascular events, such as heart attack, stroke, and cardiovascular death. The cardiovascular benefits of Ozempic are especially important for people with type 2 diabetes, who are at high risk for cardiovascular complications.
Once-Weekly Dosing: Ozempic is administered once a week by subcutaneous injection. The medication comes in a prefilled pen, allowing patients to self-administer it in the comfort of their own home. This once-weekly dosing schedule simplifies treatment and may improve compliance compared to medications that must be administered daily. Additionally, Ozempic's long-acting formulation ensures consistent glycemic control throughout the week.
Renal protection: Emerging evidence suggests that GLP-1 receptor agonists such as Ozempic may have beneficial effects on kidney function and help reduce the risk of kidney disease progression in people with type 2 diabetes. This potential kidney protection is important because kidney disease is a common complication of diabetes and a leading cause of end-stage renal failure.
Potential to reduce cardiovascular risk: In addition to reducing the risk of serious cardiovascular events,

Ozempic may also have other beneficial effects on cardiovascular health, including: B. Improved vascular function, inflammation, and lipid profile. These effects may help reduce the overall risk of cardiovascular disease in people with type 2 diabetes. Overall, Ozempic offers many benefits in diabetes treatment, including effective glycemic control, weight loss, cardiovascular benefits, ease of administration, and potential kidney protection. These benefits make it a valuable treatment option for people with type 2 diabetes who want to improve their metabolic and cardiovascular health. As with any medication, it is important for patients to discuss the potential benefits and risks of Ozempic with their doctor to determine if Ozempic is the right choice for them.

Chapter Two

DOSAGE AND ADMINISTRATION

2.1 Administration of Ozempic

Ozempic (semaglutide) is given by subcutaneous injection. Detailed instructions on how to administer Ozempic are below:

Preparation: Before administering Ozempic, it is important to wash your hands thoroughly with soap and water. Gather all necessary supplies, including the Ozempic pen, alcohol wipes, and sharps disposal container.
Choosing an Injection Site: The recommended injection sites for Ozempic are the abdomen (around the belly button), thigh, or upper arm. Choose a different injection site each week to minimize the risk of irritation or skin reactions. Prepare the injection pen: Remove

the Ozempic pen from the refrigerator and allow it to cool to room temperature for about 30 minutes before use. Do not shake the pen. Check the expiration date and visually inspect the solution for particles or discoloration. Do not use the pen if the solution becomes cloudy or discolored. Clean the injection site: Clean the injection site thoroughly with an alcohol swab. Allow skin to dry thoroughly before continuing with your injection.

Prepare the Pen Dose: Remove the cap from your Ozempic pen and insert a new sterile needle. Prepare the pen by turning the dose selector until the dose counter reads "0" and a drop of solution appears at the tip of the needle.

Adjust the Dose: Follow your doctor's instructions, adjust the dose selector to your prescribed dose. The dose selector clicks with each dose increment, allowing you to select exactly the dose you need. To inject medication: Pinch the skin fold at the clean injection site. Insert the needle into the skin at a 45-90 degree angle, depending on the thickness of the skin and the length of the needle. Press the injection button to administer the medication. Hold the button down for approximately 5 seconds to ensure the full dose is administered.

Remove the needle: After the medication has been injected, release the injection button and remove the needle from the skin. Do not rub the injection site.

Disposing of the needle: Carefully remove the needle from the pen and discard it in a needle container. Do not put the cap back on the needle.

Storage of the pen: After use, put the cap back on your Ozempic pen and store it in the refrigerator. Keep the pen from freezing and away from light. It is important to follow your doctor's instructions and Ozempic package insert carefully. If you have any questions or concerns about administering Ozempic, do not hesitate to ask your doctor or pharmacist for advice.

2.2 Injection Technique

The injection technique for Ozempic (semaglutide) follows standard subcutaneous injection procedures. Here is a step-by-step guide to the injection technique.

Preparation:

Wash your hands thoroughly with soap and water. Have all the necessary items ready, including the Ozempic pen, alcohol wipes, and needle container. Remove your Ozempic Pen from the refrigerator and allow it to cool to room temperature for about 30 minutes. Do not shake the pen. Choosing an Injection Site:

The recommended injection sites for Ozempic are the stomach (around the belly button), thigh, or upper arm. Choose a different injection site each week to minimize the risk of irritation or skin reactions.

Cleaning the Injection Site:

Wipe the injection site thoroughly with an alcohol wipe. Allow skin to dry completely before continuing with the injection.
Preparing the Injection Pen:

Remove the cap from the Ozempic Pen and attach a new sterile needle. Prepare the pen by turning the dose selector until the dose counter reads "0" and a drop of solution appears at the tip of the needle.
Setting the Dose:

Following your doctor's instructions, turn the dose selector to the prescribed dose. The dose selector clicks with each dose increment so you can select the exact dose you need. To inject medication:

Pinch the skin fold over the cleaned injection site. Insert the needle into the skin at a 45-90 degree angle, depending on the thickness of the skin and the length of the needle. Press the injection button to administer the medication. Hold the button down for approximately 5 seconds to ensure the full dose is administered.

To remove the needle:

After the medication has been injected, release the injection button and remove the needle from the skin. Do not rub the injection site.

To dispose of the needle:

Carefully remove the needle from the pen and discard it in a needle container. Do not put the cap back on the needle.

Storing the pen:

After use, place the cap back on the Ozempic pen and store in the refrigerator. Keep the pen from freezing and protected from light. It is important to follow these steps carefully and follow your doctor's instructions and the package insert for Ozempic. If you have any questions or concerns about how to inject your medicine, don't hesitate to ask your doctor or pharmacist.

2.3 Dosage Instructions

Dosage instructions for Ozempic (semaglutide) may vary based on individual patient factors and doctor recommendations. However, here are some general guidelines for dosing Ozempic:

Starting Dose: The recommended starting dose of Ozempic for most patients is typically 0.25 mg once weekly. This starting dose helps minimize the risk of gastrointestinal side effects, such as nausea and vomiting, that may occur when starting Ozempic treatment.

Titration: After 4 weeks of treatment with the initial dose, the dose of Ozempic can be increased to 0.5 mg once weekly. This dose adjustment allows patients to gradually become accustomed to the medication and reduces the possibility of gastrointestinal side effects. Maintenance dose: For many patients, the maintenance dose of Ozempic is 0.5 mg once weekly. This dose allows for effective glycemic control and weight management while minimizing the risk of side effects.

Maximum dose: For patients who need additional glycemic control, doctors may recommend increasing the Ozempic dose to 1 mg once weekly. However, this higher dose is associated with an increased risk of gastrointestinal side effects and may not be suitable for all patients.

Renal impairment: Ozempic is primarily cleared by the kidneys, so a dose adjustment may be necessary in patients with renal impairment. For patients with moderate to severe renal insufficiency, your doctor may recommend a lower starting dose and more conservative dose titration.

Missed Dose: If you miss a dose of Ozempic, it should be administered as soon as possible, but no later than 5 days after the missed dose. If more than 5 days have passed since the missed dose, skip the missed dose and take it on the next scheduled day.

Special Populations: Dose adjustments may be necessary in elderly patients, patients with hepatic insufficiency, or patients with other medical conditions that may affect the metabolism or excretion of Ozempic. Your doctor will consider individual patient factors when determining the appropriate dosage. It is important to follow your doctor's dosage instructions and the package insert for Ozempic carefully. Do not adjust your dose without first consulting your doctor. Always consult your doctor or pharmacist if you have any questions or concerns about your Ozempic dosing.

2.4 Recommended Starting Dose and Titration

The recommended starting dose and titration schedule for Ozempic (semaglutide) may vary depending on individual patient factors and your doctor's recommendations. However, here are some general guidelines for the starting dose and titration of Ozempic:

Starting Dose: The typical starting dose of Ozempic for most patients is 0.25 mg once weekly. Starting at this low dose helps minimize the risk of gastrointestinal side effects, such as nausea and vomiting, that can occur when initiating Ozempic treatment.

Titration: After 4 weeks of treatment with an initial dose of 0.25 mg once weekly, the dose of Ozempic can be increased to 0.5 mg once weekly. This titration schedule allows patients to gradually become accustomed to the drug and reduces the potential for gastrointestinal side effects.

Maintenance Dose: For many patients, the maintenance dose of Ozempic is 0.5 mg once weekly. This dose provides the benefits of effective glycemic control and weight management while minimizing the risk of side effects. It is important to note that the initial dose and titration schedule of Ozempic may be adjusted based on individual patient response, tolerability, and specific physician recommendations. Some patients may require a slower titration or a lower starting dose, especially those who are more sensitive to the drug or who have certain medical conditions that may increase the risk of side effects.

In addition, your doctor may consider factors such as renal function, hepatic function, age, and concomitant medications when determining the appropriate starting dose and titration schedule for each patient.

As always, it is important to carefully follow your doctor's dosage instructions and the Ozempic package insert. Do not adjust the dose without first consulting your doctor. Be sure to ask your doctor or pharmacist if you have any questions or concerns about starting or titrating your dose of Ozempic.

2.5 Storage Guidelines

Proper storage of Ozempic (semaglutide) is important to maintain its stability and effectiveness. Recommended storage guidelines for Ozempic are as follows:

Refrigerate: Store Ozempic in the refrigerator at a temperature between 2°C and 8°C. Store the Ozempic pen in its original packaging to protect it from light.

Do not freeze: Do not freeze Ozempic. Freezing can damage the medicine and make it less effective. Protect from light: Store your Ozempic pen in its original packaging to protect it from light. Do not expose the pen to direct sunlight or bright light for extended periods of time.

Room temperature: If needed, Ozempic can be stored at room temperature (up to 77°F or 25°C) for short periods of time up to 14 days. However, once Ozempic has been stored at room temperature, do not put it back in the refrigerator. Store at room temperature away from sources of heat, moisture, and direct sunlight. Do not use an expired pen: Check the expiration date on your Ozempic pen before using it. Do not use Ozempic if it has expired as it may no longer be effective or safe to use.

Do not shake: Do not shake your Ozempic pen. Shaking can cause air bubbles to form in the medicine, which can affect the accuracy of your dose.

Keep out of reach of children: Keep Ozempic out of reach of children and pets. If children or pets accidentally ingest Ozempic, it can pose serious health risks.

Travel: If you need to travel with Ozempic, store it in a cooler bag with ice packs to maintain the recommended temperature range. Don't leave the medication in a hot car or in direct sunlight for an extended period of time.

Following these storage guidelines is important to ensure the safety and effectiveness of Ozempic. If you have any questions or concerns about storing Ozempic, ask your doctor or pharmacist. 2.6 Proper Storage Conditions

Proper storage conditions are important to maintain the stability and effectiveness of Ozempic (semaglutide). Recommended storage conditions are:

Refrigerate: Store Ozempic in the refrigerator at a temperature between 2°C and 8°C. This is the ideal temperature range to maintain the stability of the drug.

Original Packaging: Store Ozempic in its original packaging to protect it from light. Direct exposure to light can cause the medication to degrade over time. Do not freeze: Do not freeze Ozempic. Freezing can damage the medicine and make it less effective. If Ozempic accidentally freezes, do not use it and contact your pharmacist or doctor for instructions.

Protect from heat: Do not expose Ozempic to high temperatures. Store it away from direct sunlight, heaters, radiators, and other sources of heat. Make sure room temperatures do not exceed 25°C (77°F) for any short period of time.
Avoid moisture: Keep Ozempic dry and protected from moisture. Don't store it in places where it may be exposed to water or moisture, such as in the bathroom or near a sink.
Travel: If you need to travel with Ozempic, use a portable cooler bag with ice packs to maintain the recommended temperature range while traveling. Don't leave Ozempic in a hot car or expose it to extreme temperatures for extended periods of time.
EXPIRATION DATE: Check the expiration date on your Ozempic packaging before use. Do not use Ozempic if it has expired as it may no longer be safe or effective.
Keep out of reach of children: Store Ozempic in a safe place away from children and pets. Accidental ingestion of Ozempic can cause serious injury or even death.
Following these proper storage conditions helps ensure that Ozempic remains safe and effective throughout its shelf life. If you have any questions or

concerns about storing Ozempic, ask your doctor or pharmacist.

Chapter Three

SIDE EFFECTS AND PRECAUTIONS

3.1 Common Side Effects

Ozempic (semaglutide) is generally well tolerated, but like any medicine, it can cause side effects in some people. Common side effects of Ozempic include:

Nausea: Nausea is one of the most common side effects reported by people taking Ozempic, especially when starting treatment or increasing your dose. This symptom usually improves over time as your body gets used to the medicine.

Vomiting: Some people may experience vomiting, especially during the first few weeks of treatment with Ozempic. This side effect may also lessen with continued use of the medicine.
Diarrhea: Some people taking Ozempic may experience diarrhea. It is mild to moderate in severity and usually resolves without special treatment.
Abdominal pain: Abdominal pain or discomfort may occur as a side effect of Ozempic. This symptom is usually mild and temporary. Decreased appetite: Ozempic may cause a decrease in appetite in some people, leading to reduced food intake. This effect may

contribute to weight loss, which is often desirable in people with type 2 diabetes.

Injection site reactions: Some people may experience redness, swelling, or itching at the injection site after receiving Ozempic. These injection site reactions are usually mild and go away on their own.

Headache: Headache is a common side effect of many medications, including Ozempic. Headaches with Ozempic are usually mild and temporary.

Hypoglycemia: Although less common than some other diabetes medications, hypoglycemia (low blood sugar) can occur with Ozempic, especially when taken with other blood sugar-lowering medications such as insulin or sulfonylureas. Symptoms of hypoglycemia may include sweating, trembling, dizziness, confusion, and hunger.

Constipation: Some people may experience constipation as a side effect of Ozempic. Drinking plenty of water and eating foods rich in fiber can help relieve this symptom.

Fatigue: Some people taking Ozempic may feel tired or fatigued, especially during the first few weeks of treatment. This side effect is usually temporary.

3.2 Nausea, vomiting etc.

Nausea and vomiting are common side effects of Ozempic (semaglutide), especially during the first few weeks of treatment or when the dose is increased. Here are more details on these side effects:

Nausea: Nausea is an unpleasant sensation in the stomach that may or may not lead to vomiting. It is a common side effect of many medicines, including Ozempic. Nausea with the use of Ozempic may occur immediately after administration or may last for some time. In most cases, nausea improves over time as the body gets used to the medication.
 Vomiting: Vomiting is the forceful expulsion of stomach contents through the mouth and is often preceded by nausea. Like nausea, vomiting can occur as a side effect of Ozempic, especially early in treatment. Although less common than nausea, vomiting may occur as a side effect of Ozempic in some people.
 Gastrointestinal side effects such as nausea and vomiting are thought to be due to Ozempic's effects on the gastrointestinal tract, such as delayed gastric emptying and changes in appetite regulation. In many cases, they are temporary and tend to resolve with continued use of the medication.

Here are some tips to manage nausea and vomiting associated with Ozempic:

Take Ozempic with food: Taking Ozempic with food may reduce the risk of nausea and vomiting. Eating smaller, more frequent meals throughout the day may also help.

Stay hydrated: Drink plenty of fluids, especially water, to stay hydrated. Drinking clear liquids such as water or ginger tea may reduce nausea. Avoid nausea-causing foods and smells: Certain foods, smells, or activities can cause nausea. Recognizing and avoiding these triggers can help minimize symptoms. Rest: Getting plenty of rest and avoiding strenuous activities can help relieve nausea and vomiting. Talk to your doctor: If nausea and vomiting persist or become severe, it is important to talk to your doctor. They can provide guidance on how to deal with these side effects and may recommend adjustments to your treatment plan. It's important to note that nausea and vomiting are possible side effects of Ozempic, but many people tolerate the medication well and these side effects often improve over time. If you experience persistent or severe side effects, be sure to consult your doctor so you can receive appropriate treatment.

3.3 Serious reactions

Serious reactions to Ozempic (semaglutide) are rare, but some people can experience serious side effects that require immediate medical attention. Serious reactions associated with Ozempic include:

Pancreatitis: In rare cases, Ozempic can cause pancreatitis, an inflammation of the pancreas. Symptoms include severe abdominal pain that radiates to the back, nausea, vomiting, fever and rapid heart rate. Pancreatitis requires immediate medical attention and may require hospitalization.

Allergic reactions: Although rare, some people may have an allergic reaction to Ozempic. Signs of an allergic reaction may include rash, itching, hives, swelling of the face, lips, tongue, or throat, difficulty breathing, or chest tightness. Anaphylaxis is a severe and potentially life-threatening allergic reaction that requires immediate medical attention.

Thyroid C-cell tumors: Ozempic has been associated with an increased risk of thyroid C-cell tumors in rodents. Although this risk has not been established in humans, people with a personal or family history of medullary thyroid cancer (MTC) or multiple endocrine neoplasia syndrome type 2 (MEN 2) should use Ozempic with caution and discuss the potential risks and benefits with their doctor.

Acute renal failure: Acute renal failure (AKI) has been reported in individuals receiving GLP-1 receptor agonists, such as Ozempic. Symptoms of acute kidney failure include decreased urine output, swelling in the legs and feet, fatigue, confusion, nausea, and shortness of breath. Acute kidney failure requires immediate medical attention and may require hospitalization.
Gallbladder disease: Ozempic may increase the risk of gallbladder-related side effects such as cholelithiasis (gallstones) and cholecystitis (inflammation of the

gallbladder). Symptoms of gallbladder disease include abdominal pain, nausea, vomiting, and fever.

It is important to note that severe reactions to Ozempic are possible but relatively rare. Most people tolerate the medication well and experience only mild to moderate side effects, such as nausea, vomiting, and injection site reactions. However, it is important to pay attention to signs and symptoms of severe reactions and seek immediate medical attention if they occur.

Contact your doctor or seek immediate medical attention if you experience any serious or worrying symptoms while taking Ozempic. Do not stop taking Ozempic without talking to your doctor, as suddenly stopping the medication may worsen your diabetic control.

3.4 Allergic reactions, pancreatitis, etc. Let's take a closer look at these serious reactions associated with Ozempic.

Allergic reactions:

Symptoms: An allergic reaction to Ozempic may include rash, itching, hives, swelling of the face, lips, tongue, or throat (angioedema), difficulty breathing, and chest tightness. Anaphylaxis, a severe and potentially life-threatening allergic reaction, may also occur.

Treatment: If you notice any signs of an allergic reaction, seek medical help right away. Anaphylaxis requires immediate treatment with epinephrine and emergency medical care. Pancreatitis:

Symptoms: Pancreatitis is characterized by severe abdominal pain that may spread to the back, nausea, vomiting, fever, and rapid heart rate. Treatment: If you experience symptoms suggestive of pancreatitis, such as: B. If you have severe abdominal pain, seek medical attention immediately. Pancreatitis requires immediate evaluation and treatment by a doctor, often in a hospital. Thyroid C-cell tumors: Risk: In animal studies, Ozempic has been associated with an increased risk of thyroid C-cell tumors, but this risk has not been demonstrated in humans. People with a personal or family history of medullary thyroid cancer (MTC) or multiple endocrine neoplasia syndrome type 2 (MEN 2) should use Ozempic with caution. Monitoring: Doctors may monitor people at high risk of thyroid tumors more closely during treatment with Ozempic. If you have concerns about your thyroid health, consult your doctor.
Acute Kidney Injury (AKI):

Symptoms: AKI may manifest as decreased urine output, swelling in the legs and feet, fatigue, confusion, nausea, and shortness of breath. Treatment: If you experience symptoms suggestive of AKI, see a doctor immediately. AKI requires evaluation and treatment by a doctor and may require hospitalization if severe.

Gallbladder Disease:

Symptoms: Gallbladder-related side effects such as cholelithiasis (gallstones) and cholecystitis (inflammation of the gallbladder) may manifest as symptoms such as abdominal pain, nausea, vomiting, and fever. Treatment: If you experience symptoms suggestive of gallbladder disease, contact your doctor for evaluation and appropriate treatment. It is important to be aware of these possible serious reactions associated with Ozempic and to seek immediate medical attention if you notice any symptoms suggestive of an allergic reaction, pancreatitis, thyroid tumor, acute kidney injury, or gallbladder disease. Always talk to your doctor if you have any concerns or questions about your medication.

3.5 Precautions and Warnings

Ozempic (semaglutide) is a medicine used to treat type 2 diabetes. Although it is generally safe and effective, there are precautions and warnings to be aware of when using this medicine. Important precautions and warnings associated with Ozempic include:

Pancreatitis: Ozempic has been associated with an increased risk of pancreatitis, an inflammation of the pancreas. People with a history of pancreatitis or gallbladder disease may be at higher risk. Seek immediate medical attention if you experience severe abdominal pain, nausea, or vomiting. Thyroid tumors: Animal studies have shown that taking Ozempic increases the risk of thyroid C-cell tumors. Although this risk in humans has not been established, people with a personal or family history of medullary thyroid cancer (MTC) or multiple endocrine neoplasia syndrome type 2 (MEN 2) should use Ozempic with caution.

Allergic reactions: Some people may have an allergic reaction to Ozempic that may include rash, itching, swelling of the face, lips, tongue, or throat, difficulty breathing, or chest tightness. Anaphylaxis, a severe allergic reaction, may also occur. If you notice any signs of an allergic reaction, seek medical attention immediately. Renal failure: The safety and effectiveness of Ozempic in patients with renal failure have not yet been fully established, so caution is advised when prescribing Ozempic to patients with renal failure. Dose adjustments may be necessary.
Hypoglycemia: Ozempic may lower blood sugar levels, which may increase the risk of hypoglycemia (low blood sugar). This risk may be higher when Ozempic is used in combination with other hypoglycemic medications. Monitor blood sugar levels regularly and watch for signs and symptoms of hypoglycemia. Gallbladder disease: Ozempic may increase the risk of gallbladder-related side effects, such as gallstones and gallbladder inflammation (cholecystitis). Tell

your doctor if you experience symptoms such as abdominal pain, nausea, or vomiting.

Increased heart rate: Ozempic may increase your heart rate, especially in people with existing heart disease. Caution is advised in patients with a history of cardiovascular disease or arrhythmia.

Injection site reactions: Ozempic may cause injection site reactions such as redness, swelling, and itching. Alternate injection sites and watch for signs of skin irritation or infection.

Pregnancy and breast-feeding: There is limited data on the use of Ozempic in pregnant or breast-feeding women. If you are pregnant, planning to become pregnant, or breastfeeding, consult your doctor before using Ozempic.

Hepatic Impairment: The safety and effectiveness of Ozempic in people with hepatic impairment have not been fully established, so caution is advised when prescribing Ozempic to people with hepatic impairment. Regularly perform liver function tests. Before you start taking Ozempic, it is important to discuss any medical conditions, medications, or concerns with your doctor. They will provide you with individualized advice and monitor for possible side effects while you are taking the medicine.

3.6 Special Information for Specific Populations

Special considerations for specific populations when using Ozempic (semaglutide) include:

Elderly Patients: Elderly patients may be more susceptible to certain side effects of Ozempic, such as hypoglycemia and dehydration. Doctors may consider starting at a lower dose and closely monitoring these patients for side effects.

Pediatric Patients: The safety and effectiveness of Ozempic in pediatric patients under 18 years of age have not been established. Therefore, the use of Ozempic is not recommended in this patient group.

Pregnant women: There are limited data on the use of Ozempic in pregnant women. Animal studies have shown adverse effects on pregnancy and fetal development. Therefore, Ozempic should be used during pregnancy only if the potential benefits justify the potential risks to the fetus. Healthcare providers may consider alternative treatments for pregnant women with type 2 diabetes. Breastfeeding women: It is not known whether Ozempic passes into breast milk. When using Ozempic therapy in a breastfeeding woman, doctors should weigh the potential benefits of Ozempic therapy against the potential risks to the child. Renal failure: Ozempic is primarily eliminated by the kidneys. Therefore, caution is advised when prescribing Ozempic to patients with renal failure. Dosage adjustments may be necessary in such patients. Hepatic impairment: The safety and effectiveness of Ozempic in patients with hepatic impairment have not been established. Caution is advised when prescribing Ozempic to these patients, and regular liver function testing may be required. Cardiovascular disease: Patients with a history of cardiovascular disease, such as heart failure or heart attack, should be closely monitored when using Ozempic. Although Ozempic has shown cardiovascular benefits in some studies, its use in this population should be considered with caution.

Thyroid disease: Patients with a history of thyroid disease, especially medullary thyroid carcinoma (MTC) or multiple endocrine neoplasia type 2 (MEN 2), should use Ozempic with caution. In animal studies, Ozempic has been associated with an increased risk of thyroid C-cell tumors.

Injection Site Reactions: Patients with a history of injection site reactions or skin disorders may be at increased risk of developing an injection site reaction from Ozempic. Healthcare providers should instruct patients on proper injection technique and monitor for signs of skin irritation or infection.

Drug Interactions: Ozempic may interact with certain medications, including other antidiabetic medications, increasing the risk of hypoglycemia and other side effects. Healthcare providers should review patients' medication lists and adjust dosages as needed to minimize the risk of drug interactions. It is important that health care providers take these special considerations and individual patient factors into account when prescribing Ozempic. Patients should also tell their doctor any medical conditions, medications, or concerns they have before starting Ozempic therapy.

Chapter Four

Efficacy and Clinical Studies

4.1 Clinical Studies Overview

Clinical trials are an important part of the drug development process and provide important data on the safety and efficacy of medicines like Ozempic (semaglutide). Here is an overview of the clinical trials related to Ozempic:

Phase 1 Clinical Trials: Phase 1 trials typically involve a small number of healthy volunteers and focus on evaluating the drug's safety, pharmacokinetics (how the drug moves through the body), and pharmacodynamics (how the body responds to the drug's effects). These studies help researchers determine a safe dose range for further testing.

Phase 2 Clinical Trials: Phase 2 trials involve a larger number of participants, including people with the condition the drug is intended to treat. These studies are intended to further evaluate safety and begin to evaluate the drug's effectiveness at different doses. Phase 2 trials may also explore different formulations and delivery methods.

Phase 3 Clinical Trials: Phase 3 trials are large studies involving hundreds or thousands of participants aimed at confirming the effectiveness of a drug and further evaluating its safety. These studies compare the drug to a standard of care or placebo and provide more detailed data on side effects and adverse reactions. Phase 4 Clinical Trials (Post-Marketing Surveillance): Phase 4 clinical trials take place after a drug has been approved for use by a regulatory agency, such as the FDA (Food and Drug Administration) in the United States. These studies continue to monitor the safety and effectiveness of a drug in a real-world environment and are often larger and longer-lasting than previous phases. Ozempic, in particular, has been clinically proven to be effective and safe in treating type 2 diabetes. Important clinical studies include:

The SUSTAIN clinical trial program evaluated the efficacy and safety of Ozempic in patients with type 2 diabetes. These studies showed greater reductions in HbA1c levels (a measure of blood sugar control) and weight compared to placebo and other antidiabetic drugs.

The PIONEER clinical trial program compared Ozempic to other antidiabetic drugs, including insulin and oral antidiabetic drugs. These studies showed that Ozempic was effective in lowering blood sugar levels and promoting weight loss, with a lower risk of hypoglycemia compared to insulin. Cardiovascular outcome studies (CVOTs) such as SUSTAIN-6 have examined the cardiovascular safety of Ozempic. These studies have shown that Ozempic is non-inferior to placebo in cardiovascular events and have demonstrated cardiovascular benefits in some cases.

Overall, the results of clinical trials supported the approval of Ozempic for the treatment of type 2 diabetes and provided valuable information on its safety and efficacy profile.

4.2 Summary of key studies

Here we provide an overview of some important clinical studies related to Ozempic (semaglutide) in the treatment of type 2 diabetes.

Sustain studies:

The SUSTAIN clinical trial program evaluated the efficacy and safety of Ozempic in patients with type 2 diabetes. The SUSTAIN 1-7 studies investigated various aspects of Ozempic treatment, including glycemic control, weight loss, and cardiovascular outcomes. These studies showed greater reductions in HbA1c levels and body weight compared to placebo and other antidiabetic drugs. Ozempic had a lower risk of hypoglycemia compared to insulin and was generally well tolerated.

PIONEER STUDIES:

The PIONEER clinical trial program compared Ozempic to other antidiabetic drugs, including insulin and oral antidiabetic drugs. PIONEER studies 1-9 investigated the efficacy and safety of Ozempic in different patient groups and treatment settings. Ozempic demonstrated superior or non-inferior reductions in HbA1c levels and body weight compared to other antidiabetic drugs. It demonstrated a lower risk of hypoglycemia compared to insulin and was generally well tolerated.

SUSTAIN-6 Study:

The SUSTAIN-6 study specifically investigated the cardiovascular safety of Ozempic. The study showed that Ozempic was non-inferior to placebo in cardiovascular outcomes. In addition, Ozempic demonstrated cardiovascular benefits, including reductions in major adverse cardiovascular events (MACE) and all-cause mortality compared to placebo.

SUSTAIN for Kids Study:

The SUSTAIN for Kids study evaluated the safety and efficacy of Ozempic in pediatric patients with type 2 diabetes. The studies showed that Ozempic was effective in improving glycemic control and weight loss in children and adolescents with type 2 diabetes. Ozempic was generally well tolerated in this population and had a safety profile consistent with that observed in adults. Overall, these large clinical trials demonstrated the efficacy, safety, and cardiovascular benefits of Ozempic in the treatment of type 2 diabetes. The results support its use as a valuable treatment option for patients with type 2 diabetes, providing effective glycemic control, weight loss, and reduced cardiovascular risk.

4.3 Effect on glycemic control

The efficacy of Ozempic (semaglutide) in glycemic control has been well established in various clinical studies. A summary of its efficacy is given below:

Reduction of HbA1c levels: Ozempic has consistently demonstrated a significant reduction in HbA1c levels, an important marker of long-term glycemic control, in patients with type 2 diabetes. Clinical trials have shown a 1% to 1.5% reduction in HbA1c levels compared to placebo and other antidiabetic drugs.

Reduction of fasting blood glucose levels: Ozempic is effective in reducing fasting blood glucose levels, helping to improve overall glycemic control in patients with type 2 diabetes.

Reduction of postprandial blood glucose levels: In addition to lowering fasting blood glucose levels, Ozempic also helps to reduce postprandial (after-meal) blood glucose spikes, contributing to improved overall glycemic control throughout the day. Sustained Effectiveness: Clinical studies have shown that Ozempic has long-lasting effectiveness. Continuing treatment will result in continued improvements in HbA1c levels and glycemic control.
Dose-Dependent Response: The effectiveness of Ozempic is dose-dependent. In general, increasing doses result in greater reductions in HbA1c levels and improved glycemic control. Starting at a low dose and

gradually increasing to a higher dose will optimize effectiveness and minimize the risk of side effects. Combination Therapy: Ozempic is often used in combination with other antidiabetic medications, such as metformin, sulfonylureas, and insulin, to further improve glycemic control in people with type 2 diabetes. Clinical studies have shown that Ozempic can provide additional benefits when combined with other active ingredients. Overall, Ozempic's effectiveness in glycemic control has been well established through extensive clinical studies. It offers type 2 diabetes patients an effective treatment option, helping to improve glycemic control and reducing the risk of complications associated with uncontrolled diabetes.

4.4 Lowering HbA1c Levels, Fasting Blood Glucose, and More

Of course! Let's take a closer look at the specific effects of Ozempic (semaglutide) on glycemic control, including lowering HbA1c levels, fasting blood glucose, and postprandial blood glucose.

Lowering HbA1c Levels:

HbA1c (hemoglobin A1c) is a measure of average blood glucose levels over the past 2-3 months and is an important indicator of long-term glycemic control. Clinical studies have consistently shown that Ozempic significantly reduces HbA1c levels in people with type 2 diabetes. Reductions in HbA1c levels with treatment with Ozempic were approximately 1% to 1.5%, depending on the study and patient population examined. These reductions in HbA1c levels are generally greater than those achieved with placebo or other antidiabetic drugs used as comparators in clinical trials. Improved fasting plasma glucose (FPG) levels:

Fasting plasma glucose (FPG) reflects blood glucose levels after a period of fasting and is an important measure of overall glycemic control. Ozempic was effective in reducing FPG levels in patients with type 2 diabetes, resulting in improved fasting glycemic control. Clinical studies have shown that Ozempic treatment significantly reduces FPG levels, contributing to an overall improvement in glycemic control. Lowering Postprandial Blood Glucose:

Postprandial blood glucose refers to blood glucose levels after a meal and can contribute to overall glycemic fluctuations. Ozempic has been proven to reduce postprandial blood glucose fluctuations and help stabilize blood glucose levels throughout the day. Ozempic helps lower postprandial blood glucose by slowing gastric emptying and increasing glucose-dependent insulin secretion, resulting in better overall glycemic control. Dose-Dependent Response:

The effect of Ozempic on reducing HbA1c, fasting blood glucose, and postprandial blood glucose is dose-dependent. In general, higher doses of Ozempic result in greater reductions in these parameters, with optimal effects observed with appropriate dose titration. Overall, Ozempic has demonstrated robust efficacy in improving glycemic control across multiple parameters, including reductions in HbA1c levels, fasting plasma glucose, and post-prandial plasma glucose. These effects contribute to its role as an effective treatment option for patients with type 2 diabetes.

4.5 Other Health Benefits

In addition to its primary function of improving glycemic control, Ozempic (semaglutide) has demonstrated several other health benefits that contribute to its overall effectiveness in treating type 2 diabetes. These additional health benefits include:

Weight Loss: Ozempic has been associated with significant weight loss in patients with type 2 diabetes. Clinical trials have consistently shown that treatment with Ozempic results in greater weight loss than placebo and other antidiabetic medications. The weight loss effect is thought to be due to several factors, including reduced appetite, delayed gastric emptying, and increased satiety.

Cardiovascular Effects: Ozempic has demonstrated cardiovascular benefits in patients with type 2 diabetes. Cardiovascular outcome trials (CVOTs) such as SUSTAIN-6 have found Ozempic to be non-inferior to placebo in terms of cardiovascular safety and, in some cases, have demonstrated cardiovascular benefits, such as a reduction in major cardiovascular adverse events (MACE) and all-cause death.

Lowers blood pressure: Ozempic has been shown to lower blood pressure in patients with type 2 diabetes. Ozempic helps lower blood pressure by promoting weight loss and improving overall glycemic control. This is important for reducing the risk of cardiovascular complications associated with hypertension.

Improved lipid profile: Ozempic has been associated with improved lipid profile, including lower triglyceride and LDL cholesterol levels and increased HDL cholesterol levels. These improvements contribute to a lower risk of cardiovascular events in patients with type 2 diabetes. Kidney protection: Recent evidence suggests that Ozempic may have a kidney-protective effect in patients with type 2 diabetes. Several studies have shown that treatment with Ozempic is associated with a reduction in markers of kidney dysfunction and may slow the progression of diabetic kidney disease.

Reduced risk of hypoglycemia: Ozempic is associated with a lower risk of hypoglycemia (low blood sugar) compared with several other antidiabetic medications, especially insulin and sulfonylureas. By stimulating insulin secretion and suppressing glucagon secretion in a glucose-dependent manner, Ozempic helps maintain blood glucose levels within the normal range without increasing the risk of hypoglycemia.

Overall, Ozempic offers numerous health benefits beyond its primary role of improving glycemic control, including weight loss, cardiovascular benefits, blood pressure reduction, improved lipid profile, kidney protection, and reduced risk of hypoglycemia. These additional benefits make Ozempic a valuable treatment option for patients with type 2 diabetes, especially those with comorbidities such as obesity, hypertension, dyslipidemia, and cardiovascular disease.

4.6 Weight loss, cardiovascular effects, and more

Of course! Here we consider in more detail the health benefits of Ozempic (semaglutide) on weight loss, effects on cardiovascular disease, and other relevant aspects.

Weight loss:

Ozempic has demonstrated a remarkable weight loss effect in patients with type 2 diabetes. Clinical trials have consistently shown that treatment with Ozempic results in greater weight loss compared to placebo and other antidiabetic drugs. The weight loss effect of Ozempic is thought to be multifactorial and includes reduced appetite, delayed gastric emptying, and increased satiety. On average, patients treated with Ozempic experienced a weight loss of 5-10% of their baseline body weight. This is clinically significant and may translate to improved overall health and well-being.

Cardiovascular outcomes:

Ozempic has demonstrated cardiovascular benefits in patients with type 2 diabetes. In cardiovascular outcome trials (CVOTs) such as SUSTAIN-6, Ozempic was found to be non-inferior to placebo in terms of cardiovascular safety. In addition, Ozempic demonstrated cardiovascular benefits, including a reduction in major adverse cardiovascular events (MACE), including heart attack, stroke, and cardiovascular death, compared to placebo. These cardiovascular benefits are particularly important for patients with type 2 diabetes, who are at high risk for cardiovascular complications. Lowering blood pressure:
Ozempic has been associated with lowering blood pressure in people with type 2 diabetes. Ozempic helps lower blood pressure by promoting weight loss and improving overall glycemic control. This is important for reducing the risk of cardiovascular events and other complications associated with high blood pressure.

Improved lipid profile:
Ozempic has been shown to improve the lipid profile in people with type 2 diabetes. This leads to lower triglyceride and LDL cholesterol levels and increased HDL cholesterol levels, contributing to a good lipid profile and reduced risk of cardiovascular events.

Kidney protection:
New evidence suggests that Ozempic may have a kidney-protecting effect in people with type 2 diabetes. Several studies have shown that treatment with Ozempic is associated with a reduction in markers of kidney dysfunction and may slow the progression of diabetic kidney disease.

Reduced risk of hypoglycemia:

Ozempic has a lower risk of hypoglycemia compared with some other antidiabetic drugs, especially insulin and sulfonylureas. By stimulating insulin secretion and suppressing glucagon secretion in a glucose-dependent manner, Ozempic helps maintain blood glucose levels within the normal range without increasing the risk of hypoglycemia. Overall, beyond its primary role of improving glycemic control, Ozempic offers numerous health benefits, including significant weight loss, cardiovascular benefits, blood pressure reduction, improved lipid profile, kidney protection, and reduced risk of hypoglycemia. These additional benefits make Ozempic a valuable treatment option for patients with type 2 diabetes, especially those with obesity, hypertension, dyslipidemia, and cardiovascular disease.

Chapter Five

Comparison with other diabetes medications

5.1 Comparison with insulin

When comparing Ozempic (semaglutide) to insulin, several factors must be considered, including efficacy, safety, ease of use, and side effect profile. Here is a comparison of Ozempic to insulin:

Effectiveness:

Both Ozempic and insulin are effective in lowering blood glucose levels in patients with type 2 diabetes. Ozempic acts primarily by stimulating insulin secretion in a glucose-dependent manner, inhibiting glucagon secretion, and slowing gastric emptying. Insulin directly lowers blood glucose levels by promoting glucose uptake into cells. Clinical studies have shown that both Ozempic and insulin can result in significant reductions in HbA1c levels, with Ozempic showing equal or greater efficacy in some cases. Weight loss: Ozempic is associated with weight loss, although insulin use may result in weight gain in some patients. The weight loss effect of Ozempic may be especially beneficial for overweight or obese patients with type 2 diabetes.
Risk of hypoglycemia:

Ozempic has a lower risk of hypoglycemia compared with insulin, especially when used as monotherapy or when combined with other non-insulin antidiabetic drugs. Insulin may increase the risk of hypoglycemia, especially when used in high doses or in combination with other hypoglycemic drugs.

Management:

Ozempic is administered as a subcutaneous injection once weekly, whereas insulin is typically administered as a subcutaneous injection one or more times daily, depending on the type of insulin and the individual patient's needs. Weekly administration of Ozempic may be more convenient and more reliable compared to daily insulin injections.

Side effects:

Both Ozempic and insulin can cause side effects, but the type and frequency of side effects may differ. Common side effects of Ozempic include gastrointestinal symptoms such as nausea and diarrhea, while common side effects of insulin include hypoglycemia, weight gain, and injection site reactions. Serious side effects such as pancreatitis and allergic reactions are rare but can occur with both Ozempic and insulin.

Cardiovascular effects:

Ozempic has shown cardiovascular benefits in patients with type 2 diabetes, while the cardiovascular effects of insulin are less clear. Some studies suggest that certain insulin preparations may be associated with an increased risk of cardiovascular events, especially in patients with existing cardiovascular disease.

5.2 Differences in Mechanism of Action, Efficacy, and Side Effects

Let's compare Ozempic (semaglutide) and insulin in some important aspects such as mechanism of action, efficacy, and side effects.

Mechanism of Action:

Ozempic (semaglutide):

Ozempic belongs to a class of drugs known as glucagon-like peptide-1 receptor agonists (GLP-1 RAs). It works by mimicking the action of incretin hormones, particularly GLP-1, which stimulates insulin secretion in a glucose-dependent manner, inhibits glucagon secretion, slows gastric emptying, and promotes satiety. Ozempic helps lower blood glucose levels in people with type 2 diabetes by targeting multiple aspects of glucose metabolism.

Insulin:

Insulin is a hormone produced in the pancreas that plays a central role in regulating blood glucose levels. It promotes the absorption of glucose into cells, where it can be used for energy or stored for later use. Insulin lowers blood sugar levels by promoting glucose uptake by muscle, fat, and liver cells, thereby lowering blood glucose levels. Effects:

Ozempic:
Clinical studies have shown that Ozempic is effective in lowering HbA1c levels, fasting blood glucose levels, and postprandial blood glucose fluctuations in patients with type 2 diabetes. It has also been associated with significant weight loss in many patients. The degree of HbA1c reduction with Ozempic is comparable to, and in some cases exceeds, that achieved with other antidiabetic drugs, including insulin. Insulin:
Insulin is highly effective in lowering blood sugar levels in patients with type 2 diabetes. It is particularly effective in reducing postprandial blood glucose fluctuations and controlling hyperglycemia in patients with insulin deficiency or insulin resistance. Insulin therapy can be tailored to a patient's individual needs by adjusting the dose, timing, and insulin formulation (e.g., rapid-acting, short-acting, intermediate-acting, long-acting).

Side effects:

Ozempic:

Common side effects of Ozempic include gastrointestinal symptoms such as nausea, vomiting, diarrhea, and constipation. Other possible side effects include hypoglycemia (especially when used in combination with insulin or sulfonylureas), injection site reactions, headache, and dizziness. Rare but serious side effects may include pancreatitis, allergic reactions, and kidney problems. Insulin:

Common side effects of insulin therapy include hypoglycemia, weight gain, injection site reactions (e.g., redness, swelling, itchiness), and allergic reactions (rare). Hypoglycemia is a significant risk associated with insulin therapy, especially if too much is administered or at an inappropriate time. Other possible side effects may include lipodystrophy (thickening or thinning of subcutaneous fat at the injection site), insulin resistance, and fluid retention. In summary, Ozempic and insulin have different mechanisms of action, efficacy profiles, and side effect profiles. Although both are effective treatments for lowering blood glucose levels in patients with type 2 diabetes, the choice between Ozempic and insulin depends on several factors, including individual patient characteristics, treatment goals, preferences, and tolerance to side effects. Healthcare providers should carefully consider these factors when selecting the most appropriate treatment for each patient.

5.3 Comparison with other GLP-1 agonists

When comparing Ozempic (semaglutide) with other GLP-1 agonists, several factors should be considered, including efficacy, safety, dosing frequency, and side effect profile. Below, we present a comparison with other commonly used GLP-1 agonists.

Effectiveness:

Ozempic (semaglutide):

Ozempic has shown robust efficacy in lowering HbA1c levels and fasting plasma glucose levels in patients with type 2 diabetes. It has also been associated with significant weight loss, making it particularly beneficial for patients who are obese or overweight. Other GLP-1 agonists (e.g., Victoza, Trulicity):

Other GLP-1 agonists, such as Victoza (liraglutide) and Trulicity (dulaglutide), have also been shown to be effective in lowering HbA1c levels and improving glycemic control. They may also cause weight loss, although the degree of weight loss varies with different GLP-1 agonists and individual patients.

Dosage Frequency:

Ozempic:

Ozempic is administered as a subcutaneous injection once a week. The once-weekly dosing schedule is convenient and may improve patient adherence compared to other GLP-1 agonists that require more frequent dosing.

Other GLP-1 Agonists:

Victoza is typically administered as a subcutaneous injection once a day, while Trulicity is administered once a week. Some other GLP-1 agonists, such as Byetta (exenatide) and Bydureon (extended-release exenatide), may need to be administered twice a day or once a week. Safety:

Ozempic:
Ozempic has a generally good safety profile, but common side effects include gastrointestinal symptoms such as nausea, vomiting, diarrhea, and constipation. Serious side effects such as pancreatitis and allergic reactions are rare but can occur.

Other GLP-1 agonists:
The safety profile of other GLP-1 agonists is generally similar to that of Ozempic, with gastrointestinal symptoms being the most common side effect. Some GLP-1 agonists may have specific side effects and considerations. For example, in clinical trials, Victoza has been shown to be associated with a small increased risk of pancreatitis and thyroid tumors.

Cardiovascular outcomes:

Ozempic:

Ozempic has demonstrated cardiovascular benefits in patients with type 2 diabetes, including reductions in major adverse cardiovascular events (MACE) and all-cause mortality, in cardiovascular outcomes trials (CVOTs) such as SUSTAIN-6. Other GLP-1 agonists: Several GLP-1 agonists, such as Victoza and Trulicity, have also shown cardiovascular benefits in CVOTs and reduced risk of MACE and other cardiovascular events. In conclusion, Ozempic shares similarities with other GLP-1 agonists in terms of efficacy and safety, but stands out with its once-weekly dosing schedule and proven cardiovascular benefits. The choice between Ozempic and other GLP-1 agonists depends on individual patient factors, preferences, and treatment goals and should be made in consultation with your physician.

5.4 Similarities and Differences

Safe! Let's explore the similarities and differences between Ozempic (semaglutide) and other GLP-1 agonists.

Similarities:

Mechanism of Action:

Ozempic and other GLP-1 agonists act by activating the GLP-1 receptor, which stimulates insulin secretion, inhibits glucagon secretion, slows gastric emptying, and promotes satiety. This mechanism results in

improved glycemic control, weight loss, and other metabolic effects.
Effects:

Ozempic and other GLP-1 agonists are effective in lowering blood glucose levels as measured by lowering HbA1c levels and fasting plasma glucose levels. They also promote weight loss in people with type 2 diabetes, so may be particularly beneficial in people who are overweight or obese.
Safety:

In general, Ozempic and other GLP-1 agonists have a good safety profile. Common side effects may include gastrointestinal symptoms such as nausea, vomiting, diarrhea, and constipation. Serious side effects such as pancreatitis and allergic reactions are rare but can occur with both Ozempic and other GLP-1 agonists.

Cardiovascular Benefits:

Several GLP-1 agonists, including Ozempic and other GLP-1 agonists such as Victoza (liraglutide) and Trulicity (dulaglutide), have demonstrated cardiovascular benefits in clinical trials. These cardiovascular benefits include reductions in major adverse cardiovascular events (MACE) and all-cause mortality.

Differences:

Dosing Frequency:

Ozempic is administered by subcutaneous injection once weekly, offering a convenient dosing schedule compared to other GLP-1 agonists. Other GLP-1 agonists may require daily or twice-daily injections (e.g., Victoza, Byetta), or weekly injections (e.g., Trulicity, Bydureon). Cardiovascular outcomes:

Ozempic and several other GLP-1 agonists have demonstrated cardiovascular benefits in clinical trials, but the specific outcomes and magnitude of benefit may vary by agent. For example, some GLP-1 agonists have shown reductions in specific cardiovascular endpoints, such as nonfatal heart attacks and strokes, while others may primarily reduce overall cardiovascular risk.

Side effect profile:

The general safety profile of Ozempic and other GLP-1 agonists is similar, but individual agents may have specific adverse event profiles or considerations. For example, Victoza has been shown to be associated with a small increased risk of pancreatitis and thyroid tumors in clinical trials, while other GLP-1 agonists may exhibit different risk profiles for specific side effects. In summary, Ozempic shares many similarities with other GLP-1 agonists in terms of mechanism of action, efficacy, and safety. However, differences in dosing frequency, cardiovascular outcomes, and side effect profiles may influence the choice of a different GLP-1 agonist for an individual patient. Healthcare providers should consider these factors when selecting the best treatment option for each patient with type 2 diabetes.

Chapter Six

Patient Information and Frequently Asked Questions

6.1 Patient Guidelines

Patient guidelines for the use of Ozempic (semaglutide) typically include the following recommendations:

Dosage and Administration:

Follow your doctor's dosage instructions. Ozempic is usually given as a subcutaneous injection on the same day once a week. Your doctor will determine the appropriate starting dose and may adjust the dose as needed based on your response to treatment.
Injection Technique:

Ask your doctor or pharmacist for the correct injection technique. Use a new needle for each injection and dispose of the needle properly in the needle container. Alternate injection sites to reduce the risk of injection site reactions.
Blood Glucose Monitoring:

Monitor your blood glucose regularly as directed by your doctor. Always monitor your blood glucose

levels and report any significant changes to your doctor.
Diet and Exercise:

Follow a healthy diet and exercise program as recommended by your doctor. Incorporate regular physical activity into your daily life to improve blood sugar control and overall health. Medication Adherence:

Take Ozempic exactly as prescribed by your doctor. Do not change your dosage or stop taking Ozempic without talking to your doctor.

Side Effects:

Watch for side effects of Ozempic, including gastrointestinal symptoms such as nausea, vomiting, diarrhea, and constipation. Report any side effects or unwanted reactions to your doctor right away.

Hypoglycemia:

Know the signs and symptoms of hypoglycemia (low blood sugar) and how to treat it. Be prepared to take appropriate action if you experience symptoms of hypoglycemia, such as sweating, trembling, dizziness, or confusion.

Regular follow-up tests:

See your doctor regularly to monitor your progress and adjust your treatment plan if necessary. Talk to your doctor if you have any concerns or questions about your treatment.

Prevention:

Tell your doctor about any other medical conditions you have and any other medications, supplements, or herbal products you are taking. Use caution when driving or operating machinery, especially if you experience side effects such as dizziness or blurred vision. Emergencies:

In the event of a medical emergency, such as: If you experience severe hypoglycemia or an allergic reaction, seek medical attention immediately or call emergency services. Always consult your doctor if you have any questions or concerns about using Ozempic, or if you experience any unexpected symptoms or side effects. Your doctor will give you personalized advice and support to help you manage your diabetes effectively.

6.2 Precautions, missed doses, etc.
Here you will find detailed instructions for using Ozempic (semaglutide), including information on missed doses and other considerations.

Instructions for use:

Preparing for injection:

Wash your hands thoroughly with soap and water.
Check the label on your Ozempic pen to be sure it
contains the correct medication and dosage. Remove
the cap of the pen and wipe the rubber gasket with
an alcohol swab.

Select an injection site:
Choose a clean, dry area of skin on the stomach
(abdomen), thigh, or upper arm to inject. Avoid any
areas with cuts, bruises, or inflamed areas.

Administer the injection:
Pinch the skin fold at the selected injection site.
Insert the needle into the skin at a 90 degree angle.
Press the pen button to inject the medication. Hold
the button down for at least 5 seconds to ensure the
entire dose is administered. Remove the needle from
the skin and release the needle.

Disposing of the needle:
Place the pen cap back on the Ozempic Pen.
Discard needles in needle container immediately
after use. Do not put cap back on pen or store
needle for later use.

Record of Injections:
Keep a record of each injection, including the date, time, dose, and injection site. This information will help you keep track of your medication regimen and speak to your doctor if you have concerns.

Missed Dose:
Missed Dose:
If you miss a dose of Ozempic, take it as soon as you remember, if it's within 5 days (120 hours) of the due date. If more than 5 days have passed since you missed a dose, skip the dose and take it on the next usual day. Do not take Ozempic twice on the same day to make up for a missed dose.
Adjusting your schedule:
If you regularly miss doses or have trouble remembering to take Ozempic, talk to your doctor. He or she will provide guidance on managing your medication schedule and suggest strategies to improve your adherence.
Monitoring blood sugar:
Monitor your blood sugar closely after you miss a dose of Ozempic. If your blood sugar levels change or you experience symptoms of hyperglycemia (high blood sugar), consult your doctor for further advice.
For more information:

Storage:
Store your Ozempic pen in the refrigerator at 2°C to 8°C. After use, the pen can be stored at room temperature (up to 30°C) for up to 56 days. Do not

freeze Ozempic and keep it out of direct sunlight and heat.

Travel:

When traveling, keep your Ozempic pen refrigerated in a portable cooler or insulated bag. Follow storage guidelines to ensure your medication remains effective while traveling.

Aftercare:

Make regular follow-up appointments with your doctor to monitor your progress and adjust your treatment plan if necessary. At these appointments, discuss any questions or concerns you have about using Ozempic with your doctor. Be sure to follow your doctor's instructions and the drug label when using Ozempic. If you have any questions or concerns about your treatment, don't hesitate to ask your doctor for advice or help.

6.3 Frequently Asked Questions

Here are some frequently asked questions (FAQs) about Ozempic (semaglutide) and its use in treating type 2 diabetes.

What is Ozempic and how does it work?

Ozempic is a medicine used to treat type 2 diabetes. It belongs to a class of drugs called glucagon-like peptide-1 receptor agonists (GLP-1 RAs). Ozempic works by mimicking the action of the GLP-1 hormone, which helps regulate blood sugar levels by stimulating insulin secretion, inhibiting glucagon secretion, and slowing gastric emptying.

What are the benefits of taking Ozempic? Ozempic may help improve blood sugar control, lower HbA1c levels, promote weight loss, and may also have cardiovascular benefits. It also has a lower risk of hypoglycemia than some other diabetes medications.

How is Ozempic given?

Ozempic is injected subcutaneously (under the skin) once a   week using a prefilled pen. It can be injected in the stomach, thigh, or upper arm. Can Ozempic be used alone or in combination with other diabetes medications?

Ozempic can be used as monotherapy or in combination with other antidiabetic medications such as metformin, sulfonylureas, or insulin, depending on individual patient needs and treatment goals.

What are the most common side effects of Ozempic? Common side effects of Ozempic may include gastrointestinal symptoms such as nausea, vomiting, diarrhea, and constipation. Other possible side effects may include hypoglycemia, injection site reactions, headache, and dizziness. Is Ozempic suitable for all people with type 2 diabetes?

Ozempic is not suitable for all   people with type 2 diabetes. It is important to discuss your medical history, current medications, and other health problems with your doctor before you   start   taking Ozempic.

How long does it take for Ozempic to start working?

Ozempic usually starts to lower your blood sugar levels within a few days to a few weeks of starting treatment. However, responses vary from person to person, and it may take several weeks for the drug to take full effect.

Is Ozempic covered by insurance?

Coverage for Ozempic may vary depending on your insurance plan. We recommend checking with your insurance company to see if the cost is covered and what out-of-pocket costs you may have to pay.

Can Ozempic be taken while pregnant or breastfeeding? The safety of Ozempic during pregnancy and breastfeeding has not been established. If you are pregnant, planning to become pregnant, or breastfeeding, be sure to consult your doctor before using Ozempic.

What should I do if I miss a dose of Ozempic?

If you miss a dose of Ozempic, take it as soon as you remember, as long as it is within 5 days (120 hours) of the missed dose. If more than 5 days have passed, skip the missed dose and take it on your next regular day. Do not take Ozempic twice on the same day. These are general FAQs about Ozempic, but if you have any specific questions or concerns, it is important to talk to your doctor before you start or while you are taking Ozempic.

6.4 Frequently Asked Questions

Below are some frequently asked questions and answers about Ozempic (semaglutide).

What is Ozempic used for?
Ozempic is used to treat type 2 diabetes in adults. It helps improve blood sugar control by lowering HbA1c levels and reducing the risk of hyperglycemia. How does Ozempic work?
Ozempic works by mimicking the action of the hormone GLP-1, which stimulates insulin release, inhibits glucagon release, slows gastric emptying, and promotes a feeling of fullness.
What are the most common side effects of Ozempic?
Common side effects of Ozempic may include nausea, vomiting, diarrhea, constipation, injection site reactions, headache, and dizziness.
How is Ozempic administered? Ozempic is given as a subcutaneous injection once a week using a prefilled pen. It can be injected into the stomach, thigh, or upper arm.

Is Ozempic suitable for all people with type 2 diabetes?

Ozempic is not suitable for all people with type 2 diabetes. It is important to discuss your medical history, current medications, and other health problems with your doctor before starting to take Ozempic. Can I use Ozempic alone or in combination with other diabetes medications?

Ozempic can be used as a monotherapy or in combination with other antidiabetic medications, such as metformin, sulfonylureas, or insulin, depending on individual patient needs and treatment goals.

How long does it take for Ozempic to start working?

Ozempic usually starts to lower blood sugar levels within a few days to a few weeks of starting treatment. However, individual responses may vary. Is Ozempic covered by insurance?

Coverage for Ozempic may vary depending on your insurance plan. We recommend contacting your insurance company to determine cost coverage and out-of-pocket costs.

Can Ozempic be taken during pregnancy or breastfeeding?

The safety of Ozempic during pregnancy and breastfeeding has not been established. If you are pregnant, planning to become pregnant, or breastfeeding, be sure to consult your doctor before using Ozempic.

What should I do if I miss a dose of Ozempic?

If you miss a dose of Ozempic, take it as soon as you remember, as long as it is within 5 days (120 hours) of the missed dose. If more than 5 days have passed, skip the missed dose and take your next usual dose on the next regular day. Do not take Ozempic twice on the same day. These are some frequently asked questions about Ozempic, but it's important to consult your doctor for individualized information and advice about your specific situation.

Chapter Seven

Cost and Insurance Coverage

7.1 Cost of Ozempic

The cost of Ozempic (semaglutide) may vary depending on factors such as your location, insurance coverage, dosage strength, and pharmacy prices. Without insurance coverage or assistance programs, the cost of Ozempic can be high. At the time of our last update, the average retail price for a 4-week supply of Ozempic (0.25 mg/0.5 mg/1 mg) in the United States was between $800 and $900.

However, it is important to note that many factors can affect your actual cost, including:

Insurance Coverage: If you have health insurance, your out-of-pocket costs for Ozempic may be significantly lower because your insurance company will cover a portion of your medication costs.

Pharmacy Discounts and Coupons: Some pharmacies offer discounts, coupons, or savings programs to help you reduce the cost of Ozempic. These discounts may be available through the manufacturer's website, a pharmacy's website, or a prescription drug discount card.

Manufacturer's assistance programs: Novo Nordisk, the manufacturer of Ozempic, may offer patient assistance programs or savings cards to eligible individuals to help reduce the cost of their medication. These programs may be tied to income criteria.

Generic availability: As of the last update, no Ozempic generics were available. However, if a generic version becomes available in the future, it may represent a cheaper alternative. We encourage you to check with your doctor, insurance company, or pharmacy for specific pricing information and explore options to reduce the cost of Ozempic. Additionally, if you are experiencing financial difficulties, you may be able to speak with your doctor for advice and to find an affordable treatment.

7.2 Retail Prices, Discounts, and More

The retail price of Ozempic (semaglutide) may vary based on factors such as dosage strength, quantity, pharmacy location, and available discounts and savings programs. Below is an overview of general retail prices and discounts for Ozempic in the United States.

Retail Prices: Since our last update, the average retail price for a 4-week supply of Ozempic has ranged between $800 and $900 for all available dosage strengths (0.25 mg, 0.5 mg, and 1 mg). Prices may vary by pharmacy and geographic location. Insurance Coverage:

If you have health insurance, your out-of-pocket costs for Ozempic may be significantly lower as your insurance company may cover a portion of the cost of the drug. Copayments or deductibles vary depending on your specific insurance plan and coverage level.

Manufacturer Utilities:

Novo Nordisk, the manufacturer of Ozempic, offers patient assistance programs and savings cards to eligible individuals. These programs can help reduce the out-of-pocket costs of Ozempic, especially for patients who are uninsured or underinsured. Check the manufacturer's website or contact Novo Nordisk directly for eligibility requirements and program details.

Pharmacy Discounts and Coupons:

Some pharmacies offer discounts, coupons, or savings programs for Ozempic that may lower the retail price. These discounts may be available through the pharmacy's website, prescription drug discount card, or membership program.

General Availability:

Generic versions of Ozempic are no longer available since our last update. Future availability of generic versions may provide a cheaper alternative to the brand-name drug. Recipe Savings Cards:

Some patients may be eligible for third-party prescription savings cards or discount programs. These programs can help you save even more on prescription medications, such as Ozempic. It is important to note that prices and discounts may change over time. Therefore, we encourage you to check with your doctor, insurance company, or pharmacy for the latest pricing information and available discounts for Ozempic. In addition, if you are experiencing financial difficulties, talk to your doctor, who may be able to offer assistance or suggest alternative treatment options.

7.3 Insurance Coverage

Insurance coverage for Ozempic (semaglutide) may vary depending on your specific health plan, health care provider, and individual circumstances. Here are some important points to keep in mind about Ozempic insurance coverage:

Coverage via Drug Directory:

Insurance plans typically maintain a list of covered medications, called a drug schedule. Ozempic may be included in your plan's medication schedule, but coverage may vary (e.g., preferred vs. non-preferred status). Check your plan's drug schedule or contact your insurance company to confirm coverage for Ozempic and any associated cost-sharing requirements.

Pre-authorization:

Some insurance plans require prior authorization before Ozempic or any other medications will be covered. This is when your health care provider provides information to your insurance company that certifies the medical necessity of the drug. If necessary, your health care provider's office will assist you with the approval process.

Tiered pricing:

Insurance plans often categorize medications into different tiers with different cost-sharing amounts for each tier. Lower-level medications usually have lower copayments, while higher-level medications may have higher copayments or deductibles. Ozempic may be assigned to a specific tier on your plan's drug list, which may affect your out-of-pocket costs. Coverage Limitations:

Some insurance plans may have coverage limitations, such as quantity limits or step therapy requirements for Ozempic or other GLP-1 agonists. Read your plan's policy documents or contact your insurer for coverage limitations.

Patient Assistance Programs:

If you are having difficulty affording Ozempic despite insurance coverage, you should learn about patient assistance programs offered by manufacturers or other organizations. These programs may provide financial assistance or copayment assistance to eligible individuals who meet certain criteria.

Medicare and Medicaid Coverage:

Ozempic is generally covered by Medicare and Medicaid plans, but coverage details may vary depending on the specific plan and eligibility criteria. If you have Medicare or Medicaid, contact your plan administrator or the appropriate program office to find out about coverage for Ozempic.

Appeal Procedure:

If your insurance plan denies coverage for Ozempic or imposes significant cost-sharing requirements, you have the right to appeal the decision. Your healthcare provider and patient advocacy groups can help you navigate the appeal process and advocate for coverage. To understand your potential out-of-pocket costs for Ozempic, it is important to review your insurance plan's coverage details, including the drug list, copayments, and coverage limitations. In addition, work closely with your healthcare provider and insurance company to resolve coverage-related issues and explore resources available to help you manage your medication costs.

7.4 Coverage Options, Copayment Assistance Programs

Coverage options and copayment assistance programs for Ozempic (semaglutide) can help patients obtain the medication at a more affordable price. Here is an overview of possible coverage options and assistance programs:

1. Insurance Coverage:
Health insurance plans, including private insurance, Medicare, and Medicaid, may cover Ozempic. Coverage levels and copayments may vary depending on your specific plan. Check your insurance plan's drug schedule and coverage details to determine whether Ozempic is covered and whether any associated copayments, deductibles, or deductibles are required.

2. Manufacturer Savings Programs:
Novo Nordisk, the manufacturer of Ozempic, offers savings programs and copayment assistance to eligible patients. The Ozempic Savings Card helps eligible privately insured patients save on their Ozempic prescription copayments and reduce their out-of-pocket costs to just $25 per prescription filled. Eligibility criteria, conditions and limitations apply. Patients can enroll in these savings programs

online or by calling the manufacturer's customer service line.

3. Patient Assistance Programs:

Novo Nordisk also offers patient assistance programs for uninsured or underinsured individuals who meet certain eligibility criteria. These programs provide free medications or copayment assistance to eligible patients who cannot afford their medications. Patients can apply for assistance through Novo Nordisk's Patient Assistance Programs (PAP) by submitting an application and providing proof of financial need. 4. Prescription discount cards:

Prescription discount cards, such as GoodRx, RxSaver, and SingleCare, can help you get discounts on prescription drugs like Ozempic at participating pharmacies. These cards can be used by uninsured or underinsured people to reduce the cost of their Ozempic prescriptions. Simply present your discount card when filling your prescription at the pharmacy to receive the discounted price.

5. Support from your healthcare provider:

Your healthcare provider or the staff at their office can help you choose insurance options, copay assistance programs, and prescription drug cost-reduction resources. You may have access to additional resources and patient support programs to help reduce the cost of Ozempic for eligible patients. 6. Nonprofits and Foundations:

Some nonprofits and patient advocacy groups may offer financial assistance programs or grants to help people with diabetes get the medications they need, including GLP-1 agonists such as Ozempic. Find out about available assistance programs offered by trusted nonprofits or foundations in the diabetes community. By exploring these insurance options and copayment assistance programs, patients can find ways to reduce their out-of-pocket costs for Ozempic and get their prescription medications for less. It is important to review the program details, eligibility criteria and terms before enrolling or applying for assistance.

Chapter Eight

Monitoring and Follow-Up Treatment

8.1 Monitoring Parameters

Monitoring parameters for patients taking Ozempic (semaglutide) include:

Blood Glucose Levels:

Regular monitoring of blood glucose levels is important to assess the effectiveness of Ozempic in controlling diabetes. Patients should monitor their blood glucose levels as directed by their doctor, usually by self-monitoring using a blood glucose meter. Keep a log of your blood glucose levels to track patterns and trends over time.

Hemoglobin A1c (HbA1c):

HbA1c levels are an indicator of long-term blood glucose control over the past 2-3 months. Your doctor may perform HbA1c testing periodically to evaluate the overall effectiveness of Ozempic therapy in treating your diabetes. HbA1c target levels may vary based on individual patient factors and treatment goals. Weight:

Ozempic has an effect on appetite and gastric emptying and is therefore associated with weight loss in many patients. Regular monitoring of weight can help track weight changes over time and evaluate the effect of Ozempic therapy on weight management. Renal function:

Patients with diabetes are at increased risk for kidney complications (diabetic nephropathy). Healthcare providers can monitor kidney function through tests such as serum creatinine, estimated glomerular filtration rate (eGFR), and urinary albumin excretion. Regular monitoring of kidney function is important, especially in patients with existing kidney disease or risk factors for renal complications. Liver function:

Ozempic is primarily metabolized in the liver, and liver function tests (e.g., alanine aminotransferase [ALT], aspartate aminotransferase [AST]) may be performed periodically to monitor liver health. Patients with pre-existing liver disease or risk factors for liver dysfunction may need to be monitored more closely.

Lipid profile:

Diabetes is often accompanied by dyslipidemia (abnormalities in lipid levels), such as elevated cholesterol and triglycerides. Periodic monitoring of lipid levels, including total cholesterol, low-density lipoprotein (LDL) cholesterol, high-density lipoprotein (HDL) cholesterol, and triglycerides, may be recommended to assess cardiovascular risk and determine treatment.

Blood pressure:

Hypertension is a common comorbidity in patients with type 2 diabetes and is a significant risk factor for cardiovascular complications. Regular monitoring of blood pressure and maintaining it within the recommended target range is essential to reduce cardiovascular risk.

Side Effects and Symptoms:

Patients should monitor for signs and symptoms of Ozempic-related side effects, including: B. gastrointestinal symptoms (nausea, vomiting, diarrhea), hypoglycemia, injection site reactions or allergic reactions. Report any worrisome symptoms to your doctor immediately.

Adherence to Medication and Aftercare:

Regular follow-up appointments with your doctor are
essential to   monitor progress, evaluate response to
treatment, and adjust treatment if   necessary.
Adherence to medication, lifestyle changes, and
self-management strategies should be emphasized and
supported at subsequent appointments. Patients
should work closely with their physicians to develop a
comprehensive monitoring plan tailored to their
individual needs and medical history. Regular monitoring
can   help optimize diabetes treatment and minimize
the risk of complications associated with the disease.

8.2 Recommended Laboratory Tests and Tests

The following laboratory tests and tests   are
recommended   for patients taking Ozempic
(semaglutide) for the treatment of type 2 diabetes
mellitus.

Hemoglobin A1c (HbA1c):

HbA1c reflects the average blood glucose level over
the past 2-3 months and is an   important indicator of
long-term glycemic control. HbA1c should be measured
every 3-6 months or as recommended by your
physician. HbA1c targets may vary depending on
individual patient factors, treatment goals, and
guidelines.

Fasting Plasma Glucose (FPG) or Self-Monitoring of
Blood Glucose (SMBG):

Regular self-monitoring of fasting plasma glucose
or blood glucose levels is useful to assess
short-term glycemic control. Patients may be advised to
monitor their blood glucose levels at home using a
blood glucose meter, especially when adjusting
medication dosages and lifestyle factors. Lipid
Profile:

A lipid profile test evaluates blood lipid levels,
including total cholesterol, low-density lipoprotein (LDL)
cholesterol, high-density lipoprotein (HDL) cholesterol,
and triglycerides. A lipid profile test is recommended
at least annually or depending on individual
cardiovascular risk factors and treatment goals.
Renal Function Tests:

Tests such as serum creatinine, estimated glomerular
filtration rate (eGFR), and urinary albumin-to-creatinine
ratio (UACR) evaluate kidney function. In patients with
known kidney disease, diabetes-related kidney
complications, or risk factors for kidney dysfunction,
kidney function tests are recommended annually
or more frequently.
Liver Function Tests:

Liver function tests, such as alanine aminotransferase
(ALT) and aspartate aminotransferase (AST), evaluate
liver health and function. Liver function tests may be

performed periodically to monitor for possible elevations in liver enzymes in association with Ozempic or other medications.

Blood Pressure Monitoring:

Regular blood pressure monitoring is helpful in assessing cardiovascular risk and treating hypertension. Blood pressure should be measured at each doctor's visit, and patients may be encouraged to measure their blood pressure at home between visits.

Weight and Waist Circumference:

Regular monitoring of weight and waist circumference is helpful in weight management and assessing health risks associated with obesity. Patients should be encouraged to monitor changes in weight and waist circumference over time. Side effects and symptoms:

Patients should be informed of possible side effects to Ozempic, including gastrointestinal symptoms, hypoglycemia, injection site reactions, and allergic reactions. Healthcare providers should inquire about and treat any worrisome symptoms reported by patients during return visits.

Adherence and follow-up:

Regular follow-up visits by health care providers are essential to monitor the effectiveness of treatment, adjust dosage, and address patient concerns. Follow-up visits should include assessment of medication adherence, lifestyle modifications, and self-management strategies. Individual patient characteristics, comorbidities, and treatment goals may influence the frequency and timing of certain laboratory tests and investigations. Healthcare providers should individualize monitoring plans based on patient needs and clinical judgment.

8.3 Follow-up Examinations

Follow-up visits for patients taking Ozempic (semaglutide) for the treatment of type 2 diabetes are essential to monitor treatment response, assess compliance, adjust treatment if necessary, and address any concerns or questions the patient may have. General guidelines for follow-up visits include:

Frequency of follow-up examinations:

The frequency of follow-up visits may vary based on individual patient factors, treatment response, and healthcare provider preferences. First, patients may have more frequent follow-up visits (e.g., every 1-3 months) to monitor response to treatment and adjust medication dosage. Once stable glycemic control is achieved, follow-up visits may become less frequent (e.g., every 3-6 months). Assessment of treatment response:

Healthcare providers should assess the patient's response to Ozempic therapy by reviewing glycemic control indicators such as HbA1c levels, fasting plasma glucose (FPG), and self-monitoring of blood glucose (SMBG) data. Evaluate changes in weight, blood pressure, and other relevant parameters to monitor overall health and the effectiveness of treatment.

Medication adherence:

Assess the patient's adherence to Ozempic therapy and address any barriers or challenges they may encounter. Review appropriate management techniques and assist as needed. Address any concerns or misunderstandings the patient may have regarding the medication regimen. Review lifestyle changes:

Discuss the patient's adherence to lifestyle changes, including dietary changes, physical activity, and smoking cessation efforts. Provide support, guidance, and resources to help the patient maintain a healthy lifestyle.

Monitor side effects.

Ask the patient about side effects or symptoms they have experienced since starting Ozempic therapy. Address and treat side effects promptly, and consider adjusting treatment or supportive care if necessary.

Review other medications:

Review the patient's complete medication list, including prescription and over-the-counter medications, dietary supplements, and herbal remedies. Assess possible drug interactions, side effects, and the need for medication adjustments.
Information and Advice:

Provide continuing education and counseling to help patients effectively manage their diabetes. Emphasize the importance of self-monitoring, medication adherence, lifestyle changes, and regular follow-up care.
Goal Setting and Shared Decision-Making:

Work with patients to set realistic treatment goals and develop individualized diabetes management plans. Participate in shared decision-making to reflect patients' preferences, values, and priorities.
Documentation and Communication:

Document details of follow-up appointments, including lab results, treatment adjustments, patient education, and recommendations. Communicate effectively with patients to include them in the decision-making process and ensure they understand their treatment plan.

Schedule next follow-up appointments:

Schedule next follow-up appointments to ensure ongoing monitoring and support. Provide clear instructions for when the next appointment should occur and how to contact the provider between appointments, if needed. Through regular follow-up visits, providers can optimize diabetes management, meet patient needs, and promote positive health outcomes for people taking Ozempic for type 2 diabetes.

8.4 Frequency and Purpose

The frequency and purpose of follow-up visits for patients taking Ozempic (semaglutide) for type 2 diabetes may vary depending on individual patient factors, treatment response, and physician preferences. However, general guidelines include the following:

Frequency:

Initially, patients may require more frequent follow-up visits, typically every 1-3 months, especially during the initial phase of treatment initiation and dose titration. Once stable glycemic control is achieved and the patient is tolerating the medication well, the frequency of

return visits decreases, for example, every 3-6 months.
Purpose:

Assessment of glycemic control: Evaluate the patient's response to Ozempic therapy by assessing indicators of glycemic control such as: B. HbA1c levels, fasting plasma glucose (FPG), and self-monitored plasma glucose (SMBG) data. Adjust treatment as needed to achieve and maintain target glycemic levels. Medication adherence: Assess the patient's adherence to Ozempic therapy and address any barriers or challenges that may arise in adhering to the medication plan. Emphasize proper administration techniques and provide training as needed.

Monitor for side effects.

Ask the patient about side effects or symptoms they have experienced since starting Ozempic therapy. Address and treat side effects promptly and consider adjusting treatment or supportive care as needed.

Review lifestyle changes:

Discuss the patient's adherence to lifestyle changes, including dietary changes, physical activity, and smoking cessation efforts. Provide support, guidance, and resources to help patients maintain a healthy lifestyle.

Review of Other Medications:

Review the patient's complete medication list, including prescription drugs, over-the-counter drugs, dietary supplements, and herbal medicines. Assess possible drug interactions, side effects, and the need for medication adjustments.

Education and Counseling: Provide continuing education and counseling to help patients effectively manage their diabetes. Emphasize the importance of self-monitoring, medication adherence, lifestyle modifications, and regular follow-up care.

Goal Setting and Shared Decision-Making: Collaborate with patients to set realistic treatment goals and develop an individualized diabetes treatment plan. Participate in shared decision-making to consider patient preferences, values, and priorities.

Document and Communicate: Document details of the next visit, including lab results, treatment adjustments, patient education, and recommendations.

Communicate effectively with patients, involving them in the decision-making process and ensuring they understand the treatment plan.

Schedule Next Appointment: Schedule the next follow-up appointment to ensure ongoing monitoring and support. Provide clear instructions on when to ask questions and how to contact your doctor between appointments, if necessary. Through regular follow-up visits focusing on these important aspects, doctors can optimize diabetes management, meet the needs of their patients, and promote positive health outcomes for people taking Ozempic for type 2 diabetes.

Chapter Nine

Lifestyle Recommendations

9.1 Diet and Exercise

Diet and exercise are fundamental to diabetes management and play an important role in complementing the effects of medications such as Ozempic (semaglutide). Here is how diet and exercise contribute to diabetes management:

Dietary guidelines:

Emphasis on a balanced diet that includes a variety of nutritious foods, such as fruits, vegetables, whole grains, lean proteins, and healthy fats. Limit your intake of refined carbohydrates, added sugars, saturated fats, and foods high in sodium, which may contribute to elevated blood sugar levels, weight gain, and cardiovascular risk. Promote portion control and mindful eating to manage calorie intake and promote satiety. Monitor carbohydrate intake, especially for those taking insulin or other hypoglycemic medications to regulate blood sugar levels. Carbohydrate Management:

Distribute carbohydrate intake evenly throughout the day to stabilize blood sugar levels and minimize post-meal blood sugar spikes. Choose complex carbohydrates with a low glycemic index (GI) to promote a gradual, steady rise in blood sugar levels. Consider carbohydrate counting and meal planning methods to help diabetics effectively control carbohydrate intake. Physical Activity:

Regular physical activity is important for improving insulin sensitivity, lowering blood sugar levels, promoting weight loss, and reducing cardiovascular risk. Aim for at least 150 minutes of moderate-intensity aerobic activity (e.g. brisk walking, cycling, swimming) per week, or 75 minutes of vigorous exercise divided into at least 3 days. Incorporate strength training (e.g. weightlifting, resistance bands) at least 2 days per week to build muscle mass and improve metabolic health. Encourage daily movement and reduce sedentary behavior by incorporating activities such as walking breaks, climbing stairs, and gardening. Individualized approach:

Keep in mind that dietary preferences, cultural background, socioeconomic factors, and individual lifestyle choices may influence eating patterns and exercise habits. Tailor nutrition recommendations and exercise plans to each patient's individual needs, preferences, and goals. Collaborate with a registered dietitian or certified diabetes educator to provide individualized nutrition advice and support.

Behavioral Strategies:

Provide education and support to help patients make sustainable lifestyle changes and develop healthy behaviors. Provide resources, tools, and self-management techniques to help patients make informed decisions about their diet and exercise habits. Create a supportive environment that promotes adherence to nutrition and exercise recommendations through encouragement, motivation, and accountability. By incorporating dietary changes and regular physical activity into an overall diabetes management plan, patients can increase the effectiveness of medications like Ozempic, improve blood sugar control, and reduce the risk of diabetes-related complications. Encourage patients to prioritize lifestyle changes as part of a comprehensive approach to managing their type 2 diabetes.

9.2 Importance in Diabetes Treatment

Diet and exercise are essential in diabetes treatment for the following reasons:

Blood sugar control: Both diet and exercise play an important role in controlling blood sugar levels. A healthy diet that emphasizes nutritious foods and controls carbohydrate intake helps prevent blood sugar spikes after meals. Regular physical activity improves insulin sensitivity, allowing cells to better absorb glucose from the bloodstream, helping to lower blood sugar levels.

Weight management: Maintaining a healthy weight is important to manage diabetes. Obesity is a significant risk factor for type 2 diabetes and can worsen insulin resistance. Diet and exercise are important strategies for achieving and maintaining a healthy weight. A balanced diet combined with regular physical activity promotes weight loss, prevents weight gain, and improves overall metabolic health.

Cardiovascular Health: Diabetes increases the risk of cardiovascular disease. Diet and exercise both contribute to cardiovascular health by lowering blood pressure, improving cholesterol levels, and reducing inflammation. A heart-healthy diet rich in fruits, vegetables, whole grains, and lean protein, combined with regular aerobic exercise, reduces the risk of heart disease and stroke in people with diabetes. Insulin Sensitivity: Physical activity improves insulin sensitivity, allowing cells to use insulin more effectively to regulate blood sugar levels. Regular exercise helps muscles absorb glucose from the bloodstream, reducing the body's reliance on insulin. This improves blood sugar control and reduces the need for diabetes medications, including insulin.

Manage Stress: Stress can affect blood sugar levels and make diabetes more difficult to manage. Exercise is a natural stress reliever and can help lower levels of stress hormones such as cortisol and adrenaline. Additionally, participating in enjoyable physical activity can improve mood and overall health, which can positively impact diabetes self-management.

Preventing and Treating Complications: Over time, diabetes can lead to a variety of complications, including nerve damage, kidney disease, eye problems, and foot complications. A healthy diet and active lifestyle can help prevent or delay the onset of these complications by promoting overall health and reducing the impact of diabetes on the body.

Empowerment and Self-Management: Incorporating diet and exercise into daily life can help people with diabetes take an active role in managing their disease. Making healthy food choices and exercising regularly are positive steps you can take to improve your health and well-being. This sense of empowerment translates to improved diabetes self-management and long-term health outcomes.

Overall, diet and exercise are essential parts of diabetes treatment. They work synergistically with medication and other treatments to improve glycemic control, promote overall health, and reduce the risk of diabetes-related complications. It is important for people with diabetes to work with their health care professionals to create individualized nutrition and exercise plans tailored to their needs, preferences, and medical history.

9.3 Alcohol and Smoking

Drinking and smoking can both have a significant impact on diabetes management and overall health. The impacts on people with diabetes include:

Alcohol consumption:

Moderate alcohol consumption may have health benefits, such as: B. Improving cardiovascular health and increasing insulin sensitivity. However, alcohol can have a negative effect on blood glucose levels, especially if consumed in excess or on an empty stomach. In people with diabetes, alcohol can cause hypoglycemia (low blood sugar), especially if they are taking insulin or certain medications that lower blood sugar levels. Alcohol consumption may also lead to weight gain, as alcoholic beverages are high in calories and may be accompanied by high-calorie mixers and snacks. It is important for people with diabetes to consume alcohol in moderation and closely monitor their blood sugar levels while drinking. They should also be aware of the carbohydrate content of alcoholic beverages and consider adjusting their diabetic medications and insulin doses accordingly. People with diabetes should talk to their doctor about whether it is safe for them to consume alcohol and how to drink responsibly.
Smoke:
Smoking is harmful to everyone's health, but it poses additional risks to people with diabetes. Smoking

increases the risk of cardiovascular disease, which is already elevated in people with diabetes. It can lead to heart attacks, strokes, and peripheral arterial disease. Smoking also contributes to insulin resistance, making it harder for people with diabetes to control their blood sugar. People with diabetes who smoke are at higher risk of complications such as diabetic retinopathy (eye damage), diabetic neuropathy (nerve damage), and kidney disease. Quitting smoking can significantly improve the health of people with diabetes. It can reduce the risk of cardiovascular disease, improve blood sugar control, and slow the progression of diabetes-related complications. Healthcare providers can offer smoking cessation support and resources to people with diabetes, including counseling, nicotine replacement therapy, and prescription medications. In summary, people with diabetes should be aware of the possible health effects of alcohol and smoking. Moderation and responsible choices when drinking alcohol are important, and smoking cessation is strongly encouraged to improve overall health and reduce the risk of diabetes-related complications. It is important for people with diabetes to work with their healthcare provider to develop strategies to effectively manage these lifestyle factors.

9.4 Effects on Blood Glucose and General Health

The effects of Ozempic (semaglutide) on glycemic control and general health are large and complex, contributing to its role as an effective treatment for type 2 diabetes. Here's a summary of its effects:

Glucose control:
Ozempic belongs to a class of drugs called GLP-1 receptor agonists that mimic the effects of glucagon-like peptide-1 (GLP-1), a hormone that stimulates insulin secretion and decreases glucagon secretion. This leads to improved glycemic control. Ozempic helps lower fasting and postprandial blood glucose levels by increasing insulin secretion in response to rising blood glucose levels and slowing gastric emptying. Clinical studies have shown that Ozempic is effective in lowering HbA1c levels, a measure of long-term glycemic control, when used as monotherapy or in combination with other diabetes medications. Weight loss:
In addition to its effects on glycemic control, Ozempic has been shown to promote weight loss in people with type 2 diabetes. This is thought to be due to its effect on appetite regulation and food intake. Clinical trials have consistently shown that Ozempic treatment is associated with a significant reduction in weight loss compared to placebo and other diabetes medications. It is particularly beneficial for people who are overweight or obese, as weight loss improves insulin sensitivity and metabolic health. Cardiovascular Benefits: Beyond its effects on blood glucose and weight, Ozempic has demonstrated cardiovascular benefits in type 2 diabetes patients at high risk for cardiovascular events. Clinical trials such as

SUSTAIN and PIONEER have shown that Ozempic treatment is associated with a reduced risk of major adverse cardiovascular events (MACE), including heart attack, stroke, and cardiovascular death, compared to placebo. Ozempic's cardiovascular benefits are thought to be mediated by mechanisms including improvements in blood pressure, lipid profile, and vascular function. Renal Benefits:

Emerging evidence suggests that Ozempic may have renal benefits in patients with type 2 diabetes and chronic kidney disease (CKD). Clinical studies, such as the SUSTAIN and FLOW studies, have shown that Ozempic treatment is associated with a reduction in albuminuria (urinary protein excretion), a marker of kidney damage and a risk factor for kidney disease progression. Ozempic's renal benefits may be due to its effects on blood pressure, glucose metabolism, and other factors that affect kidney function. General Health and Quality of Life:

Ozempic may contribute to the overall health and quality of life of patients with type 2 diabetes by improving glycemic control, promoting weight loss, and reducing the risk of cardiovascular and renal complications. Improved glycemic control reduces the risk of diabetes-related complications such as neuropathy, retinopathy, and nephropathy, improving long-term outcomes and reducing healthcare costs. The combination of improved glycemic control, weight loss, and cardiovascular benefits may lead to improved well-being and quality of life for people with type 2 diabetes.

Chapter Ten

Special Situations

10.1 Pregnancy and Breastfeeding

Pregnancy and breastfeeding are critical times for women with diabetes because they can have significant effects on maternal and fetal health. Key considerations for women with diabetes during pregnancy and breastfeeding include:

Pregnancy:

Preconception planning: Women with diabetes should ideally plan their pregnancy to ensure optimal glycemic control before pregnancy. Poorly controlled diabetes during pregnancy increases the risk of complications for both mother and baby.

Glycemic control: Strict glycemic control during pregnancy is essential to reduce the risk of adverse events such as miscarriage, stillbirth, congenital anomalies, macrosomia (high birth weight), and neonatal hypoglycemia.

Physician supervision: Pregnant women with diabetes should receive specialized prenatal care from a medical team experienced in managing diabetes during pregnancy. This team may include an endocrinologist, obstetrician, diabetes educator, and dietitian.

Blood sugar monitoring: Blood sugar levels should be monitored closely during pregnancy. Women may need to check their blood sugar more often than usual and aim for tight glycemic control, often at a lower target range than those who are not pregnant.

Medication adjustments: Some diabetes medications may need to be adjusted or stopped during pregnancy. Insulin is the preferred treatment for controlling blood sugar levels in pregnant women with type 1 or type 2 diabetes. Oral medications such as metformin or glyburide may be used but require careful monitoring.

Nutrition and weight gain: A balanced diet that meets the nutritional needs of both the mother and the developing fetus is important. Pregnant women with diabetes should work with a dietitian to develop a meal plan that will keep blood glucose levels within target ranges and promote adequate weight gain.

Fetal monitoring: Regular fetal monitoring, such as ultrasound scans and fetal nonstress tests, may be recommended to assess fetal growth and health.

Labor and delivery: Women with diabetes may require special care during labor and delivery, including close monitoring of blood glucose levels, administration of insulin, and interventions to prevent hypoglycemia in the newborn. Breastfeeding:

Benefits of Breastfeeding: Breastfeeding is highly recommended for women with diabetes as it provides many health benefits for both mother and baby. Breast milk is an ideal source of nutrition for infants and supports optimal growth and development.

Glucose Control: Breastfeeding may have a positive effect on the mother's blood sugar levels by increasing insulin sensitivity and aiding in weight loss after birth. However, women with diabetes should closely monitor their blood sugar levels while breastfeeding and adjust their insulin and medication dosages as needed.

Nutrition and Hydration: Lactating women need additional calories and fluids to support breast milk production. A balanced diet with nutritious foods and adequate fluid intake is essential for both the mother's health and breast milk production.
Medication compatibility: Some diabetes medications are compatible with breastfeeding, while others may require precautions or alternative options. Women should talk to their doctor about the safety of their diabetes medications while breastfeeding.
Support and education: Breastfeeding support and education are very important for women with diabetes. They can benefit from breastfeeding counseling, support groups, and resources to address common breastfeeding issues and ensure successful breastfeeding. Overall, women with diabetes should receive comprehensive prenatal care and ongoing

support during pregnancy and breastfeeding to optimize maternal and child health. Close collaboration between women, health care providers, and multidisciplinary teams is essential to ensure safe and effective diabetes management during this critical time.

10.2 Information for Pregnant or Breastfeeding People

If you have diabetes while pregnant or breastfeeding, it is important to prioritize the health of your mother and child by closely monitoring your blood glucose levels, diet, medication use, and overall health. Here are some tips for pregnant or breastfeeding people with diabetes:

During Pregnancy:

Planning before pregnancy: If possible, plan your pregnancy with your doctor to ensure optimal glycemic control before pregnancy. Proper care before pregnancy can reduce the risk of complications during pregnancy. Medical Monitoring: Seek specialized prenatal care from a medical professional experienced in treating diabetes during pregnancy. Your medical team may include an obstetrician, endocrinologist, diabetes educator, dietitian, and other specialists, as needed.

Blood Glucose Monitoring: Monitor your blood glucose closely throughout your pregnancy. Your healthcare provider will advise you on your blood glucose target levels and how often to monitor. Regular monitoring helps maintain tight blood sugar control and reduces the risk of complications for you and your baby. Medication Management: Discuss medication options with your doctor. Insulin is often the preferred treatment for controlling blood sugar during pregnancy, but other medications may be considered depending on your individual situation. Some oral medications may need to be adjusted or stopped during pregnancy. Diet: Eat a balanced diet that meets the nutritional needs of you and your baby. Work with a registered dietitian to develop a nutrition plan that maintains stable blood sugar levels and supports healthy fetal development. Monitor your carbohydrate intake and choose nutritious foods.

Weight Management: Aim for appropriate weight gain during pregnancy, as recommended by your doctor. Healthy weight gain supports fetal growth and reduces the risk of complications. Engaging in regular physical activity, as approved by your doctor, can help control your weight and improve your overall health.

Fetal Monitoring: Your doctor may recommend regular fetal monitoring, such as ultrasounds and fetal non-stress tests, to evaluate fetal growth and health. Planning for labor and delivery: Discuss your plan for labor and delivery with your doctor. You may need to take special precautions during labor to ensure optimal blood sugar control and minimize the risk of complications for you and your baby.

10.3 Renal Failure

People with renal failure (kidney disease) and diabetes require special consideration to effectively treat both conditions and minimize the risk of complications. Here are some tips for people with renal failure and diabetes.

Medical Monitoring: It is important that people with renal failure and diabetes receive specialized medical care from a health care provider experienced in treating both conditions. This may include a nephrologist (kidney specialist) and an endocrinologist (diabetologist), as well as other health care professionals as needed.

Glucose Control: For people with renal failure, maintaining stable blood sugar levels is essential to prevent further kidney damage and reduce the risk of complications such as diabetic nephropathy (kidney disease). Tight blood sugar control can slow the progression of kidney disease in some cases.
Medication Management: In people with impaired renal function, some diabetes medications may need to be adjusted or avoided due to the kidneys' reduced ability to filter and excrete drugs. These include certain oral antidiabetic medications and insulin. Your

doctor will determine the most appropriate medication regimen based on your kidney function and individual needs.

Blood Pressure Management: High blood pressure (hypertension) often accompanies both diabetes and impaired kidney function and can worsen kidney damage. Controlling blood pressure is critical to maintaining kidney function and reducing the risk of cardiovascular complications. Medications called angiotensin-converting enzyme (ACE) inhibitors or angiotensin II receptor blockers (ARBs) are often prescribed to regulate blood pressure and protect the kidneys in people with diabetes and kidney disease.

Dietary management: Follow a kidney-friendly diet that is low in sodium, phosphorus, and protein to treat kidney damage. Work with a registered dietitian to create a nutrition plan that supports both diabetes management and kidney health. You may also need to monitor your fluid intake to prevent fluid retention and electrolyte imbalances.

Fluid management: People with kidney damage may need to closely monitor their fluid intake to prevent overhydration and swelling (edema). Your doctor will advise you on how much fluid you should drink each day based on your kidney function and overall health.

Regular monitoring: Regular monitoring of kidney function, blood glucose, blood pressure and other relevant parameters is essential for people with kidney impairment and diabetes. These include blood tests, urine tests, blood pressure measurements and other tests to assess kidney function and overall health.

Smoking cessation: If you smoke, quitting is essential to protect kidney function and reduce the risk of cardiovascular complications associated with diabetes and renal insufficiency.

Exercise: Regular physical activity is beneficial for both diabetes management and overall health. However, people with kidney impairment should consult with their doctor before starting or modifying an exercise program, as certain activities may need to be modified depending on their individual health conditions and limitations.

Medication Adherence: Adhering to prescribed medication schedules is crucial to managing diabetes and kidney impairment. Take your medications as directed by your doctor and report any concerns or side effects immediately.

Overall, treating diabetes and kidney impairment requires a comprehensive approach that considers the unique challenges and risks of both diseases. Working closely with your medical team, following medical recommendations, and making healthy lifestyle choices can help you optimize your health and well-being despite this situation.

10.4 Dose Adjustments for Patients with Kidney Problems

Dose adjustments of certain medications used to treat diabetes, such as Ozempic (semaglutide), may be necessary in patients with kidney problems, such as renal impairment or chronic kidney disease (CKD). Semaglutide is primarily excreted by the kidneys, so dose adjustments may be necessary in people with renal impairment to avoid potential complications and ensure safe and effective treatment. General guidelines for dose adjustments of Ozempic in patients with kidney problems are as follows:

Physician advice: Dose adjustments of Ozempic or other medications should be made in consultation with a physician familiar with treating diabetes in patients with kidney problems, preferably a nephrologist or endocrinologist.
Assessing renal function: Doctors will assess a patient's kidney function using tests such as estimated glomerular filtration rate (eGFR) and urinary albumin creatinine ratio (UACR). These tests help determine the severity of renal impairment and determine treatment options. Dose adjustment based on eGFR: The dose of Ozempic may need to be adjusted based on the patient's eGFR, which reflects the kidneys' ability to filter waste products from the blood. If renal function declines, the dose of Ozempic may need to be reduced to prevent drug accumulation and reduce the risk of side effects. Dose adjustment guidelines: Specific

dose adjustments of Ozempic in patients with kidney problems may vary depending on the severity of renal impairment and individual patient factors. In general, the prescribing information for Ozempic includes recommendations for dose adjustments based on eGFR values. For example: For patients with an eGFR less than 30 to 60 ml/min/1.73 m2, the recommended starting dose of Ozempic may be lower and dose titration should be done with caution. Ozempic is not recommended for patients with severe renal impairment (eGFR less than 30 ml/min/1.73 sq. m) or end-stage renal disease (ESRD) requiring dialysis.

Monitoring and titration: When adjusting the dose of Ozempic in patients with kidney problems, it is essential to closely monitor kidney function and blood glucose levels. Doctors may adjust the dose based on the patient's individual response, tolerance, and changes in kidney function over time.

Consideration of other medications: In addition to Ozempic, dose adjustments may also be necessary for other diabetes medications and medications used to treat comorbid conditions in patients with kidney problems. Doctors will consider potential drug interactions and overall treatment plan when adjusting doses. Patient Education: Patients with kidney problems should be educated about the importance of medication adherence, regular check-ups, and lifestyle changes to effectively manage their diabetes and kidney disease. They are advised to be aware of signs and symptoms of possible complications and seek medical attention if any complications occur.

10.5 Hepatic Impairment

Hepatic impairment or disease can affect the metabolism and clearance of drugs such as Ozempic (semaglutide). Although semaglutide is primarily metabolized in the liver to inactive metabolites, hepatic impairment can still affect pharmacokinetics and dose adjustments may be necessary. Considerations when treating patients with hepatic impairment with Ozempic include:

Physician advice: Dose adjustments of Ozempic or other drugs should be made in consultation with a physician, preferably a hepatologist or endocrinologist familiar with treating diabetes in patients with liver disease.

Assessment of liver function: Physicians will assess a patient's liver function using tests such as liver enzyme levels (AST, ALT, ALP), bilirubin levels, and synthetic liver function markers (albumin, INR, etc.). These tests help determine the severity of liver impairment and guide treatment decisions. Dose adjustments for severity of hepatic impairment: The dose of Ozempic may need to be adjusted depending on the severity of hepatic impairment. Dose adjustments may be necessary in patients with mild to moderate hepatic impairment, while Ozempic may be contraindicated in patients with severe hepatic impairment.

 Dose adjustment guidelines: Specific dose adjustments of Ozempic in patients with hepatic impairment may vary depending on the severity of liver disease and individual patient factors. The prescribing information for Ozempic includes dose adjustment recommendations based on the Child-Pugh classification, which assesses the severity of hepatic impairment. Example:

In patients with mild hepatic impairment (Child-Pugh class A), no dose adjustment of Ozempic may be necessary. In patients with moderate hepatic impairment (Child-Pugh class B), the dose of Ozempic may need to be adjusted or the drug used with caution. Ozempic is not recommended for use in patients with severe hepatic impairment (Child-Pugh class C) due to limited data in this population. Monitoring and titration: When adjusting the dose of Ozempic in patients with hepatic impairment, close monitoring of liver function tests, blood glucose, and clinical status is essential. Healthcare providers may adjust the dose based on an individual patient's response, tolerance, and changes in liver function over time.

 Consideration of other medications: In addition to Ozempic, dose adjustments may also be necessary for other antidiabetic medications and medications used to treat comorbid conditions in patients with hepatic impairment. Healthcare providers will consider possible drug interactions and general treatment plans when adjusting the dose.

Patient education: Patients with hepatic impairment should be educated about the importance of medication adherence, regular follow-up, and lifestyle changes to effectively manage diabetes and liver disease. They are advised to be alert for signs and symptoms of possible complications and seek medical attention if any complications occur.

In general, dose adjustments of Ozempic in patients with hepatic impairment should be individualized based on the severity of liver disease, general health status, and treatment goals. Close cooperation between patients, healthcare providers, and other members of the healthcare team is essential to ensure safe and effective diabetes treatment in this patient population.

10.6 Considerations for Patients with Hepatic Impairment

Patients with liver disease, such as liver dysfunction or liver disease, should be given special attention in the treatment of diabetes, including the use of medications such as Ozempic (semaglutide). Important considerations for patients with liver problems include:

Assessment of liver function: Before starting treatment with Ozempic or any other drug, patients with liver problems should undergo a thorough assessment of liver function. These typically include blood tests to measure liver enzyme levels (e.g., ALT,

AST, ALP), bilirubin levels, and synthetic liver function markers (e.g., albumin and INR).

Determining severity: The severity of liver dysfunction will affect treatment decisions and dose adjustments. Liver impairment is often classified using the Child-Pugh grading system, which takes into account factors such as bilirubin levels, albumin levels, INR, ascites, and hepatic encephalopathy. The severity of liver impairment can range from mild to moderate to severe.

Drug selection: Some diabetes medications, such as Ozempic, may require dosage adjustments or may be contraindicated for patients with liver problems. Before prescribing Ozempic, your doctor will consider your patient's liver function and the potential risks and benefits of treatment.

Dose adjustment: Depending on the severity of liver impairment, a dose adjustment of Ozempic or other diabetes medications may be necessary. Patients with mild to moderate liver impairment may require a lower dose of Ozempic, while the drug may be contraindicated for patients with severe liver impairment. Dose adjustments are typically determined by the prescribing information and recommendations from your healthcare provider.

Monitoring: Patients with hepatic impairment should undergo regular liver function tests to evaluate the effectiveness and safety of treatment and monitor their clinical condition. Your healthcare provider may adjust the dosage of your medication over time based on changes in liver function.

Potential Drug Interactions: Patients with liver problems may take multiple medications to manage their health conditions. It is important to consider the possible interactions between Ozempic and other drugs used to treat liver disease or comorbidities. Your healthcare provider will assess the risk of drug interactions and adjust your treatment plan if necessary.

Lifestyle Modifications: In addition to drug therapy, patients with liver problems should make lifestyle changes to support their liver health and overall well-being. This includes avoiding alcohol consumption, eating a healthy diet, exercising regularly, and avoiding exposure to hepatotoxic substances.

Close Monitoring and Follow-Up: Patients with liver problems should be closely monitored and regularly followed up by their healthcare provider to ensure optimal management of their diabetes and liver disease. Healthcare providers will evaluate treatment response, monitor for possible complications, and adjust treatment plans if necessary. Overall, patients with liver problems require individualized care and treatment tailored to their unique needs and medical history. Close collaboration between patients, healthcare providers, and other members of the healthcare team is essential to achieve optimal outcomes and ensure the safety and effectiveness of diabetes treatment in this population.

Chapter 11

Conclusion

11.1 Summary of Key Points

Of course! Below we summarize key points to consider for patients with liver impairment, especially as they relate to the treatment of diabetes with medications such as Ozempic (semaglutide).

Assessment of liver function: Before starting treatment, patients with liver problems should have their liver function thoroughly evaluated through blood tests.
Determine severity: The severity of liver impairment is often classified using the Child-Pugh grading system to guide treatment decisions and dosage adjustments.
Drug choice: Some diabetes medications may require dosage adjustments or may be contraindicated for patients with liver problems. Careful consideration should be given to drug choices.
Dose adjustment: Depending on the severity of liver impairment, dosage adjustments of medications such as Ozempic may be necessary to ensure safety and efficacy. Monitoring: Regular monitoring of liver function tests and clinical status is essential to assess the effectiveness and safety of treatment.

Potential for drug interactions: Patients with liver impairment may be at risk for drug interactions and therefore should have their medication regimen carefully evaluated.

Lifestyle changes: Lifestyle changes such as avoiding alcohol and eating a healthy diet, as well as other health benefits, are important to support liver health in patients with liver problems.

Close monitoring and follow-up: Regular follow-up appointments with a healthcare provider are necessary to monitor the effectiveness of treatment and adjust the treatment plan if necessary.

By considering these important points and providing individualized care, healthcare providers can effectively manage diabetes in patients with liver problems while minimizing potential risks and complications.

11.2 Future Developments

Future developments in diabetes treatment, including the use of agents such as Ozempic (semaglutide), are likely to include several promising areas of research and innovation. Future developments to consider include:

Advances in GLP-1 receptor agonists: Continued research into GLP-1 receptor agonists such as semaglutide may lead to the development of new formulations with improved efficacy, safety, and ease of use. This could include longer-acting formulations and alternative delivery methods, such as oral or buccal administration.

Personalized medicine approaches: Integrating personalized medicine approaches, such as genetic testing and biomarker analysis, could help tailor diabetes treatment to patients' individual needs. This could include identifying genetic markers and metabolic profiles that are predictive of response to specific agents such as Ozempic. Combination Therapies: Combination therapies targeting multiple pathways involved in diabetes pathophysiology may result in greater efficacy and better outcomes. Future developments may explore combinations of GLP-1 receptor agonists with other classes of antidiabetic drugs, such as SGLT-2 inhibitors and DPP-4 inhibitors, to improve glycemic control and achieve additional benefits, such as weight loss and cardiovascular protection.

Gene Therapy and Regenerative Medicine: New technologies in gene therapy and regenerative medicine have the potential to treat the underlying causes of diabetes and restore pancreatic function. Future developments may include gene editing techniques to correct genetic mutations associated with diabetes and transplantation of stem cell-derived insulin-producing cells.

Digital Health Solutions: The integration of digital health technologies, such as wearable devices, mobile apps, and telehealth platforms, could revolutionize diabetes management by enabling real-time monitoring, personalized feedback, and remote access to medical experts. Future developments may focus on enhancing the usability, accuracy, and accessibility of these digital health solutions for patients with diabetes.

Artificial Intelligence and Predictive Analytics: Artificial intelligence (AI) and machine learning algorithms have the potential to analyze large datasets and identify patterns that can inform personalized treatment decisions and predict future health outcomes for patients with diabetes. Future developments may involve the integration of AI-driven predictive analytics into clinical practice to optimize diabetes management strategies.

Long-Term Safety and Outcomes Data: Continued research into the long-term safety and outcomes associated with GLP-1 receptor agonists, including Ozempic, will provide valuable insights into their role in diabetes management and their potential effects on cardiovascular health, renal function, and other important clinical endpoints.

Patient Empowerment and Education: Future developments in diabetes management will likely emphasize patient empowerment and education, empowering individuals with diabetes to take an active role in their care through self-monitoring, self-management, and informed decision-making. This includes innovative educational resources, support networks, and behavioral interventions to promote sustainable lifestyle changes and improve health outcomes.

Overall, future developments in diabetes management promise to improve outcomes, patient experiences, and expand our understanding of this complex metabolic disease. By fostering innovation and collaboration across specialties, healthcare professionals can work toward more effective, personalized, and holistic approaches to diabetes care.

Made in United States
Troutdale, OR
01/28/2025

28417485R00076